1999

PHYSICIAN PROFILING

THE CENTER FOR RESEARCH IN
AMBULATORY HEALTH CARE ADMINISTRATION

PHYSICIAN PROFILING

A Source Book for Health Care Administrators

Edited by

Neill F. Piland

Kerstin B. Lynam

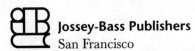

Jossey-Bass Publishers
San Francisco

Jossey-Bass books and products are available through most bookstores. To contact Jossey-Bass directly, call (888) 378–2537, fax to (800) 605–2665, or visit our website at www.josseybass.com.

Substantial discounts on bulk quantities of Jossey-Bass books are available to corporations, professional associations, and other organizations. For details and discount information, contact the special sales department at Jossey-Bass.

 Manufactured in the United States of America on Lyons Falls Turin Book. This paper is acid-free and 100 percent totally chlorine-free.

Library of Congress Cataloging-in-Publication Data

Physician profiling : a source book for health care administrators / Neill F. Piland, Kerstin B. Lynam, editors.
      p. cm.
    Includes bibliographical references and index.
    ISBN 0-7879-4601-X (hc : alk. paper)
    1. Physician practice patterns. I. Piland, Neill Finnes.
II. Lynam, Kerstin.
    [DNLM: 1. Physician Practice Patterns. 2. Data Collection.   W
87 P579 1999]
    RA399.A1P497   1999
    362.11068'5—dc21
    DNLM/DLC
    for Library of Congress   99-11319
                                     CIP

FIRST EDITION
HB Printing 10 9 8 7 6 5 4 3 2 1

CONTENTS

THE EDITORS

Neill F. Piland is research director at the Center for Research in Ambulatory Health Care Administration. He has been project director on the Robert Wood Johnson Foundation-sponsored Physician Profiling Study; co-investigator on the Physician Compensation and Risk-Bearing Arrangements in Medical Groups Project, with the University of Washington School of Public Health; and principal investigator on studies funded by ASTRA Merck and IMS America dealing, respectively, with capitation in gastroenterology practices and the marketplace for medical groups.

Kerstin B. Lynam is the contract and grants officer for the Center for Research in Ambulatory Health Care Administration (CRAHCA) and serves as the project manager on several CRAHCA publications. In addition, she performs fiscal grant management and budgeting functions for CRAHCA's research projects and operates as the fiscal administrator for other CRAHCA activities.

THE CONTRIBUTORS

E. Andrew Balas is director of the Center for Health Care Quality and Thomas P. Weil Distinguished Professor in the School of Medicine at the University of Missouri. He also serves on the faculty of the Executive Program of the National Center for Managed Health Care Administration and the Medical Informatics Training Program of the National Library of Medicine. He has developed quality improvement projects for leading health care organizations nationwide and has designed several innovative information systems.

Suzanne Austin Boren is a senior research specialist with Health Management and Informatics, School of Medicine, University of Missouri-Columbia. Her professional experience in health care project development emphasizes the areas of continuous quality improvement, clinical process management, and research methodology. She has published several articles in the areas of health care research methodology, quality improvement, and medical informatics.

Peter Braun, a consultant to the Codman Group, is a retired lecturer in the Department of Health Policy and Management at the Harvard School of Public Health. He has been involved in a variety of developments, including new applications of relative value units in provider profiling, detection of fraud and abuse, and the development of indicators to support disease management. He was coprincipal investigator of the studies of resource-based relative values of physicians' services in the United States that led to Medicare physician payment reform in 1992.

Donna L. Burman is the research database administrator at the Center for Research in Ambulatory Health Care Administration. Her primary responsibilities include application and database optimization, performance, and maintenance of the overall integrity of the CRAHCA Physician Profiling Project database.

Philip Caper is an adjunct lecturer on health policy and management at Harvard University's School of Public Health and an associate in health policy and management at the School of Hygiene and Public Health, Johns Hopkins University. He is also chairman and CEO of the Codman Group, a software and consulting firm whose cost and quality management initiatives are based on innovative statistical analyses of administrative and clinical data. An internationally recognized expert on medical care costs and quality, he has written extensively about health policy and planning and has been directly involved in the policy and planning processes.

Douglas A. Conrad is a professor in the Department of Health Services, School of Public Health and Community Medicine, and Department of Dental Public Health Sciences, School of Dentistry, and adjunct professor, Department of Finance and Business Economics, School of Business Administration, of the University of Washington, Seattle. His current research examines physician compensation models in physician group practices, conceptual development and actual behavior of integrated health systems, and the performance of community care networks in the United States. His most recent book is *Managed Care Contracting: Concepts and Applications for the Health Care Executive* (1996). In June 1996 he was named an AHSR Fellow by the Board of the Association for Health Services Research in recognition of his work in health services research. He currently serves on the editorial board of *Health Services Research.*

Philip L. Cyr is a senior research analyst at HCIA, Inc., Response Products Division, which provides software and analytic tools to measure patient-centered outcomes. His research interests include the use of data from patient satisfaction and health status surveys to predict health care expenditures.

Norbert Goldfield is an internist with a subspecialty in adolescent medicine and medical director for 3M Health Information Systems. In this capacity, he has worked on a number of projects, including the development of the outpatient prospective payment system recently passed by Congress, development of risk adjusters for episodes of illness, refinement of severity-adjusted diagnosis-related groups, and new methods of measuring quality of care. He has published extensively. He is editor of the *Journal of Ambulatory Care Management* and of *Physician Profiling and Risk Adjustment* (1999).

Ralph Insinga is a research assistant at the Medical School of the University of Wisconsin at Madison. He was a 1997–98 Fulbright scholar and served as a visiting research associate at the United Nations Economic Commission for Latin America and the Caribbean in Santiago, Chile.

Kui Chun Su is a research fellow with Health Management and Informatics, School of Medicine, University of Missouri-Columbia. She has professional expertise in biomedical literature search and research experience in systematic review, meta-analyses, database design, abstracting and indexing, experimental design, data collection and management, survey validation, and statistical analysis of data in the areas of health care quality and medical informatics.

Beth Marie Landon has been active in health affairs since the early 1990s when she developed and implemented behavior change interventions for ethnic minorities in Thailand with the Peace Corps. Since then she has worked in the areas of rural community health needs assessments, youth tobacco prevention, managed care consultancies, behavior change intervention consultancies, international HIV/AIDS networks, and international finance related to maternal and child health. She currently is active in women and children's health issues.

Daniel W. Malloy is vice president of the Managed Care and Pharmaceutical Division of HCIA, a health care information management company that specializes in outcome measurement, provider profiling, custom studies and systems, and data warehousing. HCIA works with health plans, integrated delivery systems, and pharmaceutical companies to operationalize quality improvement and disease management programs. He served as chair of the Audit Committee for the national report card project of the National Committee for Quality Assurance (NCQA), the original demonstration project for using the Health Plan Employer Data and Information Set to assess health plan performance. He is a frequent contributor to national forums on performance measurement and quality improvement, including serving as a faculty member for NCQA.

Jay Noren is vice chancellor for health affairs and president of the Health Science Center of the Texas A&M University System. He was one of the originators and former director of the graduate program in administrative medicine at the

University of Wisconsin. He started the Wisconsin Center for Health Policy and Program Evaluation and has served as vice chancellor for health sciences at the university and chancellor of Minnesota State Colleges and Universities. His research interests are physician compensation issues, managed care, the role and operation of academic health centers, Native American health care, Medicaid health maintenance organizations, analysis of primary care practice, and the physician workforce. He has also served as president of the Association of Teachers of Preventive Medicine and as visiting faculty in the Department of Health Services at the University of Washington.

Theresa A. Ryan-Mitlyng is medical director of the Lehigh Valley Physician Group, a large multispecialty group practice affiliated with Lehigh Valley Hospital, Allentown, Pennsylvania. She serves as one of three physician members on the national board of the Medical Group Management Association and on the Education Advisory Committee for the Center for Education in Medical Practice Management, which is the source for all educational development and programming for MGMA, the Center for Research in Ambulatory Care Administration, and the American College of Medical Practice Executives educational programs. With Christine Micklitsch she coauthored *Physician Performance Management: Tools for Survival and Success* (1995).

Anne Sales is an assistant professor in the Department of Health Services, School of Public Health and Community Medicine, University of Washington, Seattle, and a research scientist in the Health Services Research and Development Field Program at the Veterans Administration Puget Sound Health Care System, Seattle. Her research activities have focused on issues related to health care workforce supply and demand.

Norman S. Smith is a senior health economist for the CSC Healthcare Group, and has been working closely with the faculty at the Johns Hopkins University on case mix adjustment methodologies and the development and implementation of the Johns Hopkins ACG Case-Mix System. He has been involved with health care organizations for twenty years.

Manon Spitzer Ruben is vice president for applications development at the Codman Group. She has led the group's efforts to develop and apply morbidity assessment and risk adjustment techniques to population-based studies, provider profiling activities, network evaluation and management, and detection of health care fraud and abuse.

Robin M. Thibodeau is a research assistant for the Center for Research in Ambulatory Health Care Administration, the research and development arm of the Medical Group Management Association. Her professional experience is in health services and clinical outcomes research. At CRAHCA, she has worked on numerous research projects related to group practice, including managing the breast cancer outcomes assessment study, assessment of geriatric case management models in multispecialty groups, and the study of managed care issues in group practices.

Zung Vu Tran is a senior research scientist for the Center for Research in Ambulatory Health Care Administration. He is also professor (adjunct) of pediatrics at the University of Colorado Health Sciences Center. He has participated in all aspects of the research enterprise, both as principal investigator and as co-investigator in NIH-funded projects. In addition, he served as the senior statistician on CRAHCA's physician profiling project. He has considerable expertise in multivariate statistics and computer-intensive statistical techniques and is best known for his work in meta-analysis. His publication record includes more than sixty research papers covering a broad spectrum of biomedical interests.

Jim Tufano is a research project manager and consultant with the Department of Health Services, School of Public Health and Community Medicine at the University of Washington, Seattle. His main research interests are the nature and impact of financial incentives in medical group practices, technology assessment, and informatics and decision sciences.

To my children, Evan, Spencer, and Arden,
who have made it all worthwhile
Neill F. Piland

To my parents, Gisela and Hans Bogena,
who taught me that ethics apply to all we do
Kerstin B. Lynam

PREFACE

P*hysician Profiling* is one of the key tools to quantify quality health care delivery services. With the increase of managed care and competition to provide health care service cost-effectively, health administration professionals need to understand how profiling can best support their operations. The book intends to educate health care administrators and physician managers to ask the right questions to start and maintain their profiling systems. The following chapters address profiling development processes from initial needs assessment to implementation of lessons learned from analysis. Guidance on which data are needed for physician profiles, developing evidence-based profiling, and the use of profiling data to determine physician compensation are presented in an easy to understand, practice-oriented manner. In addition to the intrinsic challenges of implementing and using a profiling system, the book also addresses practice management issues as how to use profiling as a change agent—to turn analysis into action.

As a collective work, the book draws on the experiences of physician profiling users, developers, and researchers alike. The book presents the academic research foundation while continuously linking theory to the practical needs of medical group practices.

April 1999
Englewood, Colorado

Neill F. Piland
Kerstin B. Lynam

INTRODUCTION: THE STORY OF PROFILING

Zung Vu Tran, Donna L. Burman

For nearly three decades the health care industry has worked on developing systems designed to bring control and accountability to the delivery of health services. These systems have focused on health care utilization and costs and health care quality. A number of different mechanisms have been designed and implemented to control the effects of provider decisions on the cost and quality of care.

Such utilization review techniques as prior authorization and concurrent review, most often undertaken at the administrative or third-party payer level, are aimed at discrete and easily identifiable services or physician orders. Typically, however, they exhibit substantial shortcomings in achieving the goals of either quality assurance or cost containment. The major problem is that the system's end point is usually denial of payment for services already performed. Therefore the real or opportunity cost of care have already been incurred, and the resources used for the care have already been expended. Therefore, only the distribution of the additional costs is left to be determined. In addition, these mechanisms are inadequate to illuminate the quality of care provided. There are few guidelines and even fewer benchmarks on which to base an evaluation of care.

Although these mechanisms are still in use, the situation began to change in the mid-1980s as major integrated health care systems and third-party payers began to adopt some Continuous Quality Improvement (CQI) and Total Quality Management (TQM) techniques. These techniques, which required the generation of longitudinal performance data, performance guidelines, and benchmarking information, were applied to the areas of patient care quality and outcomes as well as resource utilization.

One of the major evaluation techniques generated by this process is that of physician or, more generally, provider profiling, with profiles generated for clinical and economic performance evaluation and improvement. Profiling is a particularly promising accountability and quality improvement instrument because it has great potential as an educational tool. Sources of variation in practice patterns are identified, quantified, and communicated to providers in an effort to reduce unnecessary variation and rationalize the delivery process. In this manner, providers actively participate in systematic efforts to modify their care-related behavior.

Profiling, which is also performed for economic purposes and can be used by delivery and insurance systems as mechanisms to control costs, is a potentially powerful evaluation and educational tool that can be developed further and made substantially more sophisticated. Certainly it will evolve at an increasing rate as health care information systems and evaluation methodologies improve.

Profiling is the collection, analysis, and use of provider practice data using epidemiological methods (McNeil, Pedersen, and Gatsonis, 1992). More specifically it is the concept of focusing on and analyzing patterns of care rather than specific clinical decisions (Lasker, Shapiro, and Tucker, 1992). The practice pattern of a single physician or a group of physicians is often expressed as a rate that incorporates some measure of resource use (costs or services) or outcome (functional status, morbidity, or mortality) that is measured over a defined period for the population served (Lee, Shapiro, Lasker, and Bindman, 1992). Physician profiling systems that focus on quality improvement gather information about practice patterns through individual feedback, peer comparison, face-to-face communication, and continuous programming to increase the understanding of the costs of overused services (Goldfield, 1996).

The following methodological criteria are important if the profiling information is to be valid (Shapiro, Lasker, Bindman, and Lee, 1993):

- Profiles must be analyzed for a well-defined population.
- A sufficient number of observations should be included to be sure that differences are not due to chance (that is, the analysis should have adequate statistical power).
- Adjustments should be made for differences in case mix.
- Profile analyses should be based on a small enough organizational unit so that members within this unit will feel responsible for the results and can work as a group to identify necessary corrective actions.

All things considered, it is difficult to make valid judgments regarding practice styles, for several reasons. First, observations (data) based on administrative or billing data sets may not have been rigorously collected and thus subjected to sampling and other errors. Second, little is known about what constitutes "average" or even "desirable" behavior nationally. Generally only the practice styles or profiles of local physicians are accessible for comparison. Finally there is the variation in the type of patients being treated. These factors have made it difficult to establish typical practice styles for purposes of profiling (Welch, Miller, and Welch, 1994). Profile development is complicated by the fact that practice-based norms, once they are available, do not necessarily reflect clinically appropriate medical care. Standards-based norms, to the extent that they are based on sound practice guidelines that are grounded on scientific evidence, can reflect appropriate care (Physician Payment Review Commission, 1992).

To profile physician performance with valid results is a difficult, time-consuming process. Nevertheless, the development and transmittal of physician-level performance measures is an important component of the effort to improve the efficiency and effectiveness of the health care delivery system.

Why Profile Physician Work?

Competitive and financial pressures on medical group practices continue to increase. The pressure to change is understandable given that health care delivery systems, specifically medical practices, tend to organize themselves according to the way providers are paid (Sandier, 1989). Practices' responses to market pressure are focused on a variety of strategic goals. In some markets, health care organizations are placing an increased emphasis on primary care on the service delivery side. In other markets, increased managed care and capitated payments on the financial side tend to focus activities on resource allocation within the systems. The medical practices across the country that have not yet addressed these issues nevertheless recognize that pressures to change will eventually affect them. In any case, given the current and predicted changes in the health care delivery systems, most practices recognize the need to understand resource use within the organization, manage available resources more efficiently, and better understand practice patterns within the practice and how these patterns compare to peer groups.

One of the challenges for practices that are preparing or already responding to market pressures is the need for information that allows them to examine resource utilization and practice patterns. In a fee-for-service setting, financial and administrative data may be sufficient to manage practices. However, in an increasingly competitive and managed care market, it is important to integrate financial, administrative, and clinical information to document quality of care and to lower costs through more appropriate utilization, to make more efficient use of providers, and to reduce practice variations. With these kinds of data, practices can better understand aspects of utilization and patterns of care.

Resource utilization, in terms of types of care, location of care, provider of care, technologies used, and other factors, is an important determinant of the cost of health care. Estimates are that physicians and osteopaths are directly or indirectly responsible for 70 percent of all health care expenditures (Knickman and Thorpe, 1990). Thus, physicians' roles in resource utilization combined with competitive market forces exert pressure on practices to define and measure physician work efforts and link these work efforts to clinical practice outcomes for resource utilization management (Brueggemann, Clark, and Ling, 1995).

Approaches to Physician Profiling

The typical approach to physician profiling is to present the same type of statistics for the profiled physician and a peer group of participating physicians with comparable demographics (such as specialty, years in practice, and gender). Observations are made on several quality or performance indicators to determine whether the comparisons indicate an outlying pattern of practice—that is, one significantly different between the performance of the profiled physician and the peer group performance.

If the profile shows that the physician is a performance outlier, he or she is presented with a more detailed analysis of data to identify possible reasons that this physician's utilization is outside the norm. Data based on only a few cases may be imprecise and thus disregarded. Or it may be that the physician–peer group differences can be traced to imprecise or inaccurate (diagnosis or procedure) coding, which may then be remedied through discussion with the responsible physician or office staff. A more substantive pattern of care that deviates from peer standards would more likely result in some intervention that is directed not only to the manner in which the physician provides services, but also to the overall management of care and perhaps the choice of specialists for referral.

Physicians themselves have recognized the appeal of profiling and feedback when they are placed at financial risk for the utilization of services. For example, a survey of ninety-four medical group practices in California (with a total of 2.9 million capitated patients) that contract with a health maintenance organization found that 79 percent of these groups profile individual physician utilization rates, with 58 percent reporting these results to their physicians (Kerr and others, 1995). Most also used profiling of utilization patterns (79 percent), guidelines (70 percent), and managed care education (69 percent). Of the fifty-four groups reporting utilization profiles to their physicians, 61 percent never adjusted for case mix among patients and more than 60 percent suggested practice changes to their physicians based on utilization. Fewer than 35 percent of the groups surveyed used written guidelines for expensive tests that required preauthorization (such as angiography). Kerr and others concluded that physicians were responding to capitation by using utilization management techniques that previously only insurers used.

Use of Claims and Other Administrative Data in Profiling

Weiner and others (1995) attempted to demonstrate that claims data profiling can be used as an ongoing method to support ambulatory care quality improvement. They based a cross-sectional study on a 100 percent sample of the Medicare claims (Part B and Part A) submitted between July 1, 1990, and June 30, 1991. Data were collected from all primary care practices (both solo and group) actively seeing patients with diabetes in Alabama, Iowa, and Maryland ($n = 2,980$). The elderly (age sixty-five years or greater) Medicare patients were seen by the study physicians and assigned a diagnosis of diabetes ($n = 97,388$) by any office-based physician during the year. Based on analyses of services provided in the ambulatory setting, these researchers found that 84 percent of diabetics did not appear to receive the recommended hemoglobin measurement, 54 percent did not see an ophthalmologist, and 45 percent received no cholesterol screening. Practice pattern profiles varied considerably across the three states (up to nearly two and a half times), even after adjusting for patient case mix and physician characteristics. The study concluded that elderly patients with diabetes do not appear to be receiving optimal care. This study underscores the value of physician profiling and practice guideline development and dissemination in the ambulatory arena. These data provide evidence that existing administrative claims data can be used to support ambulatory quality improvement activities.

Chang and McCracken (1996) conducted a study with two primary objectives: (1) to develop a simple and meaningful performance efficiency index for profiling primary care physician practice patterns and (2) to test the explanatory power of the ambulatory care group case mix system in controlling for variation in patients' resource needs. The findings indicate that large administrative databases can provide valuable information for health services management. The findings also indicate that efforts should be made to focus on methodological issues in analyzing the data sources. Conventional demographic risk-adjustment factors (age and sex) are not adequate. Greater priority needs to be given to developing and applying additional risk-adjustment systems to maximize the value of large administrative databases in profiling the relative efficiency of primary care physicians.

To provide a concrete example of profiling, Welch, Miller, and Welch (1994) analyzed the inpatient practice patterns of physicians in Florida and Oregon. They used data for 1991 from Medicare's National Claims History File to profile 12,720 attending physicians in Florida and 2,589 in Oregon. The total relative value of each physician's services delivered during each patient's hospital stay was determined. Relative value was measured in relative-value units (RVUs), according to the Resource-Based Relative-Value Scale (RBRVS) Medicare uses in determining payments to physicians. The mean number of RVUs per admission was then adjusted for the physician's case mix according to the patients' assigned diagnosis-related groups. The influence of the physician's specialty and selected types of services (such as imaging and endoscopy) was also examined. Results showed that, on average, Florida physicians used more resources than their colleagues in Oregon (46 versus 30 case-mix-adjusted RVUs per admission), with the difference consistent across all specialties and all types of service. Specific data on individual physicians and for various types of service for staffs of three hospitals were also examined. Despite similar overall profiles that fell below the national mean, each staff had a different practice pattern and would require different interventions to improve efficiency.

The authors concluded that profiling data help identify and characterize differences in practice style to which individual physicians or hospital staffs can respond. Profiling is not a well-defined and specific process. Thus, it is a cost-containment strategy that is preferable to methods where the appropriateness of each clinical decision is judged separately.

Determining the Success of Physician Profiling

Whether done by a health care plan or a medical group practice, the effects on resource utilization of profiling physicians have received relatively little rigorous investigation. Following is a review and summary of the literature concerning physician profiling and resource utilization. Most of the studies reviewed fall into three areas of resource utilization by physicians: length of hospital stay, use of tests, and drug prescription.

Length of Stay

Johnson and Martin (1996) examined the effectiveness of a physician profiling program targeting elective total hip replacement in reducing consumption of hospital resources. Over seven weeks, verbal and written data were provided to individual surgeons that profiled their own practice and those of their peers. Results showed that the length of hospital stay for patients receiving total hip replacement dropped significantly from 13.7 days to 9.9 days, and adjusted total charges dropped from $22,103 to $18,607. The variance for length of stay and total charges also dropped by at least 50 percent each.

Evans, Hwang, and Nagarajan (1995) analyzed the effectiveness and implications of introducing patient length-of-stay profiles to physicians at a hospital. Data from twenty-four thousand patients treated by four hundred physicians in 450 diagnosis-related groups over forty-two months were analyzed, including both pre-profiling and postprofiling periods. The objective was to determine whether more physicians achieved the length-of-stay benchmark after profiling was introduced, controlling for physician, disease category (diagnosis-related group), and patient severity level. Results showed a significant increase in the percentage of physicians who achieved the length-of-stay benchmark after the introduction of profiling. Physicians who initially failed to meet the benchmark reduced their patients' average length of stay much more than the physicians who initially achieved the benchmark.

Further, reductions occurred primarily at intermediate disease severity levels and in diagnosis-related groups with a large economic impact for the hospital. This profiling program appeared to achieve the objective of decreasing resource utilization by reducing patient length of stay. However, an analysis of monthly data on total weighted procedures showed that the reduction in length of stay was associated with an increase in the number of procedures performed per patient-day.

Utilization of Laboratory Tests

Ramoska (1998) analyzed the effect of information sharing through physician profiling on resource utilization of emergency room physicians. In a pre- and post-audit of laboratory use in a community hospital, a nine-month control period was followed by a fifteen-month period in which data on physicians' laboratory utilization were presented and discussed at monthly meetings. Results showed that laboratory use decreased by 17.8 percent, from a mean of 2.4 tests per patient during the control period to 1.9 during the final quarter of the study. Actual laboratory costs per month decreased by 17.7 percent, from a mean of $32,415 per month to $26,687. In addition there were no adverse changes to other quality improvement indicators. Thus, it appears that information-sharing profiling can affect resource utilization by decreasing the number and cost of laboratory tests that emergency physicians order without an adverse change in routine quality improvement indicators.

Berwick and Coltin (1986), in a cross-over study, tested three interventions to determine their impact on the rate of utilization of twelve commonly ordered blood

tests and roentgenograms among internists in a health maintenance organization. During a sixteen-week period, individual physicians received confidential feedback concerning their rates of resource utilization compared with peers (cost
feedback). Overall use of tests decreased by 14.2 percent, with eleven of the twelve
tests showing some decreases. Similar feedback on rates of abnormal test results
(yield feedback) and a program of test-specific education did not show a consistent
effect. Variability in test utilization rates (measured by the coefficient of variation)
decreased by 8.3 percent with cost feedback, 1.3 percent with yield feedback, and
2.3 percent with education. However, these decreases were inconsistent across tests.

Marton, Tul, and Sox (1985) compared two interventions by assigning fifty-six
medical house officers to four groups: a control group; a feedback group that
received feedback concerning its use of tests; a manual group, which received a
manual concerning cost-effective laboratory use; and a manual plus feedback group,
which received both interventions. All intervention groups experienced significant decreases in test use. When controlled for diagnosis, the manual plus feedback
group showed the largest decrease (42 percent) in laboratory utilization, followed
by the manual group. The feedback and control groups showed no changes. Two
interventions (manual and manual plus feedback) appeared to be effective in decreasing house staff utilization of the outpatient laboratory.

To test methods of promoting routine cancer screening, sixty-two internal
medicine residents were randomly assigned to receive cancer screening reminders
(computer-generated lists of overdue tests at patients' visits), audit plus feedback
(monthly seminars about screening, with feedback about their performance rates),
or a no intervention control group (McPhee, Bird, Jenkins, and Fordham, 1989).
Half of the residents in each group also were randomized to receive patient
education (the patients received literature and notices of overdue tests). Samples
of each physician's medical records were reviewed to determine performance
on seven tests during nine-month periods before and after the interventions.
The cancer screening reminders increased performance on six of seven tests, audit
plus feedback on four of seven tests, and patient education on one of two targeted
breast cancer screening tests. These results indicate that the cancer screening
reminders strategy was the most effective in promoting the performance of routine cancer screening tests.

Williams and Eisenberg (1986) conducted a controlled trial to evaluate a program to decrease the unnecessary utilization of inpatient testing by medical residents at a university medical center. The program used education, concurrent
feedback, and resident participation in program planning. Using specific criteria
for 7,891 chart audits of patients who had repeat tests within seven days, the investigators measured change in testing among forty-four first-year residents and forty-
three second-year residents. There were no significant differences related to the

program. It was concluded that substantial overuse of diagnostic tests did occur, that it varied from hospital to hospital, and that the program could not overcome powerful counteracting influences. Future studies, using control groups and chart audits, should evaluate interventions other than education.

In an institutional quality assurance program in hypertension, performance of tests, control of blood pressure, and follow-up were monitored through a computer program developed to audit records in an automated record system (Winickoff, Wilner, Neisular, and Barnett, 1985). Two types of feedback were provided on a quarterly basis for a one-year period to providers in the intervention group. When all hypertensive patients were analyzed together, no differences were seen between providers' scores in the intervention and control groups. The scores were based on the percentage of patients meeting preset criteria on testing, 87 percent versus 87 percent; blood pressure control, 58 percent versus 59 percent; or follow-up, 79 percent versus 77 percent. In a subanalysis of moderate to severe hypertensives, small but significant group differences did occur. Thus, interventions designed to deal with patients whose blood pressure was uncontrolled appear to be more effective than those whose blood pressures were high-normal.

Eisenberg and others (1977) developed a computer-based system to detect inappropriate utilization of laboratory resources and test a program to reduce physician resource utilization. The hospital laboratory's computerized reporting system was modified to identify patients with three or more determinations of lactic dehydrogenase (LDH) or calcium during the preceding seven days. These patients' charts were then audited to determine whether multiple tests were justified. During the control period, 51 percent of the charts audited for multiple determinations of LDH showed overutilization. During the study period, when physicians were notified if overutilization was detected, 65 percent of the charts showed overutilization. This difference (51 percent versus 65 percent) was not statistically significant. A simultaneous, undisclosed audit of calcium determinations also showed no changes between the two periods. This intervention, consisting of notification and education of physicians, was not effective in reducing overutilization of laboratory resources.

Eisenberg (1977) evaluated the effectiveness of an educational program in decreasing utilization of the prothrombin time determination by house staff physicians at a teaching hospital. Six months after the intervention, use of the prothrombin time determination as a routine admission test had decreased significantly, from 87 percent to 55 percent. Eighteen months later, however, use of this test by the physicians had returned to initial levels. These results emphasize the need to measure the long-term outcomes of interventions aimed at changing the clinical behavior of physicians and the importance of instituting follow-up programs to ensure that intervention efforts will have a lasting effect.

Utilization of Pharmacy Resources

In a prospective controlled trial, Frazier and others (1991) determined whether an intervention program featuring a drug cost manual can help physicians reduce their patients' out-of-pocket prescription drug expenses. The study took place in a general internal medicine–teaching clinic at a university hospital. Fifty-one medical interns took part, with thirty-one receiving a manual of comparative drug prices annotated with prescribing advice, two utilization feedback reports, and weekly cost-oriented prescribing reminders. The remaining interns served as the control group and concurrently were given a manual-based educational program on cholesterol management.

Over an eight-month period, 3,012 prescriptions were analyzed for cost information using a coding scheme devised by the authors. Within a given drug class, a score of 3 was assigned to the most expensive, a 2 was assigned to the intermediate-priced, and a 1 was assigned to the least expensive drug or drugs in that class. Results showed that physicians in the intervention group, compared to the control group, prescribed significantly less expensive drugs within classes of drugs. In addition, an increased supply of medication was dispensed per prescription, thereby reducing dispensing fees. This intervention appeared to help physicians reduce their patients' drug expenses and thus their own resource utilization.

Lassen and Kristensen (1992), in another prescription-based study, intervened using peer comparison feedback and the encouragement of local peer group discussions. Fifty-three medical group practices were assigned to the intervention group and fifty-five to the control group. Data for this study, based in Denmark, were obtained from computerized registration of prescriptions. The investigators found that during the six-month study period, the median costs per prescription increased significantly in the control group, whereas no statistically significant change in the intervention group occurred. There were no significant effects on the amount of drugs prescribed in either group.

Parrino (1989) developed an automated peer comparison feedback method to profile physician utilization of pharmacy resources. Since antibiotics account for an increasing percentage of hospital pharmacy charges, a one-year experiment was conducted to examine hospital antibiotic utilization. Each month attending physicians in the upper fiftieth percentile for pharmacy expenditures were notified of their status in relation to their peers. Expenditures for intervention (feedback) and control groups were compared to determine whether feedback would result in reduced expenditures by individual physicians, or whether there would be a general reduction in expenditure by the entire group. In this study, automated profiling through peer comparison feedback was not an effective method for reducing antibiotic utilization.

Steele, Bess, Franse, and Graber (1989) conducted a prospective, randomized, controlled trial, based in a Veterans Administration hospital general medicine clinic, to compare the cost-effectiveness of two interventions designed to reduce physicians' resource utilization (drug-prescribing costs). Physicians were randomized to one of three groups. Pharmacists visited one group of eleven physicians weekly to detail the prescribing of certain targeted drugs. A second group of ten physicians was given data each week comparing individual prescribing costs to those of their colleagues (peer comparison feedback profiling). The third group of ten physicians served as a control and received neither intervention. Both intervention groups received written, patient-specific suggestions for cost-effective prescribing.

Baseline prescribing costs were monitored through the hospital's computer system over a three-month preintervention period and a seven-month intervention period. The 2,026 written suggestions made by the pharmacists resulted in 613 (30.3 percent) prescribing changes: deletion, substitution, or changes in dosage of targeted drugs. There were no differences between the two intervention groups in their responses to the written suggestions. However, in comparison to the control group, the group receiving face-to-face visits from the pharmacists had lower prescription costs for seven of the eight months of the intervention. Using face-to-face meetings was cost-effective, saving $478 per physician over seven months. Since there was no significant decrease in the number of prescriptions written by the face-to-face group compared to the control group, drug substitution rather than deletion appeared to have been used by physicians to lower overall drug costs. No cost savings resulted from the use of peer comparison feedback. Thus, to reduce physicians' prescribing costs, personal visits by pharmacists are cost-effective and superior to peer comparison feedback.

Other Measures of Utilization

Pugh and others (1989) examined the effect on charges using daily charge feedback. Sixty-eight house staff physicians and sixteen teaching attending physicians participated in a controlled trial over a thirty-five-week period. During this time, 1,057 patients were under these physicians' care. There were no significant differences in charges when all patients were included in the analysis. However, since the house staff had no chance to influence 45 percent of the patients who had planned protocol admissions (diagnostic workups or protocol treatment), these patients were excluded in a subsequent subgroup analysis. In this analysis, significant reductions in total charges (17 percent), length of stay (18 percent), room charges (18 percent), and diagnostic testing (20 percent) were found. Thus, charge feedback appears to be effective in decreasing resource utilization (charges).

Reid and Lantz (1977) studied twenty-one members of a graduate internal medicine training program to determine whether feedback of simple ambulatory practice profiles would prove valuable in their training program. Each physician was profiled every three months with regard to number of patients seen, average cost of ancillary testing per visit, average time per visit, and success at obtaining patient compliance. Patients treated by both groups of physicians were similar in characteristics. Physicians were randomly selected to receive or not receive profiling reports. Variation among physicians' productivity and resource utilization ranged from 250 percent to 1,200 percent. The distribution of profiling reports did not significantly affect costs, time, or number of patients seen but did correlate with an increase in patients' compliance. The rather large variation in physicians' performances suggested that attention to style of practice during physicians' training could produce a significant increase in the amount of services delivered for each health dollar consumed.

Winickoff, Coltin, Morgan, and Buxbaum (1984) evaluated physician performances in colorectal cancer screening as part of an ambulatory quality assurance program. During a three-and-a-half-year period, three different intervention strategies for improved compliance with specific practice standards were sequentially implemented and assessed: (1) educational meeting, (2) retrospective feedback of group compliance rate, and (3) retrospective feedback of individual compliance rate. Individual physicians' profiles were compared to their peers, and a pretest-posttest design was used to evaluate the first two interventions. Neither resulted in significant improvement in compliance. Monthly feedback of individual performance compared to that of peers was then implemented in a randomized clinical trial using a crossover design. During the first six-month period, physicians receiving feedback (group 1) improved from 66.0 percent to 79.9 percent compliance; the control group (group 2) also improved, from 67.5 percent to 76.6 percent, suggesting a spillover effect.

During the second six-month period, group 2 received feedback, and group 1 did not. Group 1 stabilized at approximately 80 percent compliance, while group 2 continued to improve, from 76.6 percent to 84.0 percent. Behavior changes persisted at six and twelve months postintervention.

Summary of Results

The results of physician profiling as it affects different measures of resource utilization are mixed. The studies that measured the effects of profiling differ by type of physicians profiled (specialties, although most were family and general practice), setting (hospital, group practice), intervention (peer comparison, informational), frequency (daily, weekly to every three months), study design (uncontrolled,

controlled), and measures of resource utilization (number of laboratory tests, total charges, costs, number of prescriptions). Qualitatively there do appear to be overall, if modest, reductions in resource utilization as a result of the application of these varied interventions. However, without a rigorously designed and carefully performed study aimed specifically at the quantification of effects, it is difficult to address the overall efforts of profiling.

An important consideration in assessing the validity of the results, especially in this area of research, is the study design. Although uncontrolled studies can and do produce valuable information, research in areas where the desired outcome is a behavioral change is particularly vulnerable to threats to internal validity. Without a comparison or control group, it is difficult to determine whether it is the intervention, the act of participating in a study (the so-called Hawthorne effect),[1] or a combination of the two that produces the observed change. Thus, the results of controlled studies should be examined carefully and carry more weight than results of uncontrolled ones.

In addition to considerations related to study design is the problem of determining the overall direction and magnitude of the profiling effect on physician behavior (resource utilization). Since the results of the published research are varied, with some studies showing significant improvement in resource utilization and others showing none, meta-analysis would be particularly useful as a quantitative tool to synthesize the results of these studies. One such meta-analysis exists: that by Balas and others (1996). These investigators addressed the problems of mixed results and internal validity by using only controlled trials in examining the effects of physician profiling on resource utilization. Thus, threats to internal validity were minimized, increasing the confidence of the interpretation of the results and conclusions of the review.

Twelve studies met their inclusion criteria, which encompassed prospective, contemporaneously controlled clinical trials with random assignment to the groups (intervention, control), peer comparison feedback intervention designed to change the average utilization of a specific procedure, and outcomes measured as the frequency of a clinical activity or procedure (Berwick and Coltin, 1986; Frazier and others, 1991; Hershey, Goldberg, and Cohen, 1988; Lassen and Kristensen, 1992; Marton, Tul, and Sox, 1985; McPhee, Bird, Jenkins, and Fordham, 1989; Pugh and others, 1989; Reid and Lantz, 1977; Steele, Bess, Franse, and Graber, 1989; Winickoff, Coltin, Morgan, and Buxbaum, 1984; Winickoff, Wilner, Neisuler, and Barnett, 1985; Wones, 1987). The overall results of this meta-analysis were disappointing: there was a statistically significant but quite modest effect of peer comparison feedback on the utilization of the various clinical procedures under study, favoring the profiled groups. From this, Balas and others (1996) concluded that the "potential cost-saving effect of peer comparison feedback is unlikely to exceed the cost of the intervention for most clinical procedures." Further, they said, "Peer comparison feedback alone cannot be considered a substantive quality improvement or cost-control intervention," and it is "unfortunate that profiling of physicians has become common practice before being strongly supported by numbers in randomized controlled clinical trials" (p. 588). However, here again this conclusion stems from studies that meet very strict inclusion criteria and may represent some bias in reporting. Studies specifically designed to address this question need to be performed.

The Future of Physician Profiling

The primary goal of physician profiling should be the development of information useful to clinicians and clinical managers in evaluating practice patterns (Goldfield, 1996). Primary emphasis should be placed on demonstrating the effectiveness of the care, not the efficiency of the production. It is possible to produce unnecessary and potentially harmful services in a very efficient manner. The restoration or improvement of patients' functional health status should constitute the real outcome of the care (Kazandjian, 1996).

It seems relatively evident that the application of physician profiling data through informal peer comparison feedback by itself produces a relatively weak effect. More substantive feedback (see, for example, Ramoska, 1998) and other methods of information intervention need to be developed to improve the quality of health care and control costs through appropriate utilization of resources. These results must be rigorously evaluated.

Current concerns for small sample sizes, validity of methods for risk adjustment, and reliability of data collection methods along with other methodological concerns have resulted in mixed opinions regarding physician profiling as a tool for improving quality of care (Massanari, 1994). However, in the light of pressures for health care reform and skepticism regarding health plan and third-party payers' ability to make adequate health care policy decisions, it is unlikely that methodological concerns will dissuade major players in health care from expanding scrutiny of physician practice patterns.

Conclusion

Many of the physician profiling questions and concerns raised by the research summarized in this chapter are addressed in this book: new and better techniques of measurement and reporting in areas of resource use, clinical outcomes, quality of life, overall patient care outcomes, and patient satisfaction. This is a rapidly evolving field that is both a driver and is driven by advances in information technology and management. As the demand for accountability in health care increases, so will the use of physician profiling. It will be increasingly apparent that decisions must be based on a solid research evidence foundation. Once this is established and the implications of profiling are fully understood, progress toward valid and useful systems will be rapidly made.

Note

1. The need for control groups in social and behavioral research became clear in connection with studies of employee satisfaction conducted in the late 1920s and early 1930s by Roethlisberger and Dickson (1939). A series of experiments were performed concerning working conditions in the telephone bank wiring room at the Western Electric Hawthorne Works in Chicago. The objective was to discover what changes in working conditions would improve employee satisfaction and productivity. To the investigators' satisfaction, they discovered that making working conditions better consistently increased satisfaction and productivity. For example, as the work room was brightened through better lighting, productivity went up. Lighting was further improved, and productivity went up again. To validate their conclusions, the investigators then dimmed the lights. Productivity again improved. It became evident that the wiring room workers were responding more to the attention that the investigators gave them than to the improvements in working conditions.

References

Balas, E. A., and others. "Effect of Physician Profiling on Utilization: Meta-Analysis of Randomized Clinical Trials. *Journal of General and Internal Medicine*, 1996, *11*, 584–590.

Berwick, D. M., and Coltin, K. L. "Feedback Reduces Test Use in a Health Maintenance Organization." *Journal of the American Medical Association*, 1986, *255*, 1450–1454.

Brueggemann, J. G., Clark, T. C., and Ling, G. "Physician Work Effort RVUs: Use in a Multispecialty Group Practice." *Group Practice Journal*, 1995, *44*, 26–30.

Chang, W., and McCracken, S. B. "Applying Case Mix Adjustment in Profiling Primary Care Physician Performance." *Journal of Health Care and Finance*, 1996, *22*, 1–9.

Christiansen, C. L., and Morris, C. N. "Improving the Statistical Approach to Health Care Provider Profiling." *Annals of Internal Medicine*, 1997, *127*, 764–768.

Eisenberg, J. M. "An Educational Program to Modify Laboratory Use by House Staff." *Journal of Medical Education*, 1977, *52*, 578–581.

Eisenberg, J. M., and others. "Computer-based Audit to Detect and Correct Overutilization of Laboratory Tests." *Medical Care*, 1977, *15*, 915–921.

Evans, J. H. III, Hwang, Y., and Nagarajan, N. "Physicians' Response to Length-of-Stay Profiling." *Medical Care*, 1995, *33*, 1106–1119.

Frazier, L. M., and others. "Can Physician Education Lower the Cost of Prescription Drugs? A Prospective, Controlled Trial." *Annals of Internal Medicine,* 1991, *115,* 116–121.

Goldfield, N. "Profiling and Quality Improvement: Concluding Remarks, 1996." In N. Goldfield and P. Boland (eds.), *Physician Profiling and Risk Adjustment.* Gaithersburg, Md.: Aspen.

Hershey, C. O., Goldberg, H. I., and Cohen, D. I. "The Effect of Computerized Feedback Coupled with a Newsletter upon Outpatient Prescribing Charges: A Randomized Controlled Trial." *Medical Care,* 1988, *26,* 88–94.

Johnson, C. C., and Martin, M. "Effectiveness of a Physician Education Program in Reducing Consumption of Hospital Resources in Elective Total Hip Replacement." *Southern Medical Journal,* 1996, *89,* 282–289.

Kazandjian, V. A. "Public Disclosure: A Hospital Quality Improvement Project's Perspective, 1996." In N. Goldfield and P. Boland (eds.), *Physician Profiling and Risk Adjustment.* Gaithersburg, Md.: Aspen.

Kerr, E. A., and others. "Managed Care and Capitation in California: How Do Physicians at Financial Risk Control Their Own Utilization?" *Annals of Internal Medicine,* 1995, *123,* 500–504.

Knickman, J. R., and Thorpe, K. E. "Financing for Health Care." In A. Kover (ed.), *Health Care Delivery in the United States* (pp. 240–269). New York: Springer, 1990.

Lasker, R. D., Shapiro, D. W., and Tucker, A. M. "Realizing the Potential of Practice Pattern Profiling." *Inquiry,* 1992, *29,* 287–297.

Lassen, L. C., and Kristensen, F. B. "Peer Comparison Feedback to Achieve Rational and Economical Drug Therapy in General Practice: A Controlled Intervention Study." *Scandinavian Journal of Primary Health Care,* 1992, *10,* 76–80.

Lee, P. R., Shapiro, D. W., Lasker, R. D., and Bindman, A. B. "Managed Care: Provider Profiling." *Journal of Insurance Medicine,* 1992, *24,* 179–181.

Marton, K. I., Tul, V., and Sox, H. C., Jr. "Modifying Test-Ordering Behavior in the Outpatient Medical Clinic: A Controlled Trial of Two Educational Interventions." *Archives of Internal Medicine,* 1985, *145,* 816–821.

Massanari, R. M. "Profiling Physician Practice: A Potential for Misuse." *Infection Control and Hospital Epidemiology,* 1994, *15,* 394–396.

McNeil, B. J., Pedersen, S. H., and Gatsonis, C. "Current Issues in Profiling Quality of Care." *Inquiry,* 1992, *29,* 298–307.

McPhee, S. J., Bird, J. A., Jenkins, C. N., and Fordham, D. "Promoting Cancer Screening: A Randomized, Controlled Trial of Three Interventions." *Archives of Internal Medicine,* 1989, 149, 1866–1872.

Parrino, T. A. "The Nonvalue of Retrospective Peer Comparison Feedback in Containing Hospital Antibiotic Costs." *American Journal of Medicine,* 1989, *86,* 442–448.

Physician Payment Review Commission. *Conference on Profiling.* Washington, D.C.: PPRC, May 1992.

Pugh, J. A., and others. "Effect of Daily Charge Feedback on Inpatient Charges and Physician Knowledge and Behavior." *Archives of Internal Medicine,* 1989, *149,* 426–429.

Ramoska, E. A. "Information Sharing Can Reduce Laboratory Use by Emergency Physicians." *American Journal of Emergency Medicine,* 1998, *16,* 34–36.

Reid, R. A., and Lantz, K. H. "Physician Profiles in Training the Graduate Internist." *Journal of Medical Education,* 1977, *52,* 301–307.

Roethlisberger, F. J., and Dickson, W. J. *Management and the Worker.* Cambridge, Mass.: Harvard University Press, 1939.

Rosen, A. K., Houchens, R. L., Gibson, T. B., and Mayer-Oakes, A. "Developing Episodes of Care for Adult Asthma Patients: A Cautionary Tale." *American Journal of Medical Quality,* 1998, *13,* 25–35.

Salem-Schatz, S., Moore, G., Rucker, M., and Pearson, S. D. "The Case for Case-Mix Adjustment in Practice Profiling: When Good Apples Look Bad." *Journal of the American Medical Association,* 1994, *272*(11), 871–874.

Sandier, S. "Health Services and Utilization of Physician Income Trends." *Health Care Financing Review,* 1989, Annual Supplement, 32–48.

Shapiro, D. W., Lasker, R. D., Bindman, A. B., and Lee, P. R. "Containing Costs While Improving Quality of Care: The Role of Profiling and Practice Guidelines." *Annual Review of Public Health,* 1993, *14,* 219–241.

Spoeri, R. K., and Ullman, R. "Measuring and Reporting Managed Care Performance: Lessons Learned and New Initiatives." *Annals of Internal Medicine,* 1997, *127*(Pt. 2), 726–732.

Steele, M. A., Bess, D. T., Franse, V. L., and Graber, S. E. "Cost Effectiveness of Two Interventions for Reducing Outpatient Prescribing Costs." *DICP Annals of Pharmacotherapy,* 1989, *23,* 497–500.

Weiner, J. P., and others. "Variation in Office-Based Quality: A Claims-Based Profile of Care Provided to Medicare Patients with Diabetes." *Journal of the American Medical Association,* 1995, *273,* 1503–1508.

Welch, H. G., Miller, M. E., and Welch, W. P. "Physician Profiling: An Analysis of Inpatient Practice Patterns in Florida and Oregon." *New England Journal of Medicine,* 1994, *330,* 607–612.

Williams, S. V., and Eisenberg, J. M. "A Controlled Trial to Decrease the Unnecessary Use of Diagnostic Tests." *Journal of General and Internal Medicine,* 1986, *1,* 8–13.

Winickoff, R. N., Wilner, S., Neisuler, R., and Barnett, G. O. "Limitations of Provider Interventions in Hypertension Quality Assurance." *American Journal of Public Health,* 1985, *75*(1), 43–46.

Winickoff, R. N., and others. "Improving Physician Performance Through Peer Comparison Feedback." *Medical Care,* 1984, *22*(6), 527–534.

Wones, R. G. "Failure of Low-Cost Audits with Feedback to Reduce Laboratory Test Utilization." *Medical Care,* 1987, *25*(1), 78–82.

PHYSICIAN PROFILING

PART ONE

METHODOLOGY

CHAPTER ONE

LAYING THE FOUNDATION FOR A PROFILING SYSTEM

Norman S. Smith

The development of a practice profiling system in the medical group requires three basic elements: (1) identification of the types of information that would be most useful to the group, which can easily differ from medical group to medical group; (2) setting priorities to determine which aspects will be developed first, which includes recognizing immediate limits, including those imposed by data availability; and (3) gaining commitment for the resources necessary to developing or implementing the system.

A practice profiling system and information that will allow better management of patients and practice finances by the administrator, individual physicians, and other service providers can be extremely important. Some aspects of profiling can be implemented only at the medical group level—for example, the history of immunizations or family history. The medical group is the only place where targeted historical data on patients can be gathered about patients for practice profiling purposes; no one else will be able to gather this information and develop profiles on other aspects of patient and provider behavior and interaction for some time to come.

On the other hand, external data are vital for profiling some of the aspects of a practice that may be the most important. Practices accepting global risk cannot have any idea of measuring performance without access to detailed information, at least at the claim or encounter level, supplied by all providers of care who interact with their patients. If a medical group is at risk for the costs of hospitalizations or for referrals outside the practice, detailed data on these aspects at the encounter level must be made available if practice management is to improve. If the practice is losing money on risk-related contracting, for example, no one may know, without substantial external data, whether practice managers need to work with individual physicians to show them better ways to provide necessary care or to find a way to recruit and retain less risky patients.

There are at least as many different physician profiles as there are organizations preparing them. These profiles, usually provided by integrated delivery networks, hospitals, health maintenance organizations (HMOs), or other insurance carriers, include various permutations and combinations of information on financial performance, patient satisfaction, quality in all of its guises, outcomes, conformance to established protocols, certifications, incidence of malpractice suits, and the like. These are typically compilations of raw information unadjusted for the types of patients being served or the specific nature of the practice. When physicians are involved in the design of profiling systems, information is more likely to be adjusted for age and sex to make reports more comparable. Other techniques including morbidity-based population adjustment and episode adjustment tools are being demanded by physicians and their administrative staffs.

At some point in the not-so-distant future, the success and survival of individual medical groups will very likely depend on their ability to access data and turn them into the management information contained in a comprehensive profiling system. Physicians and medical group administrators who recognize this need will be successful; those who do not will be less likely to succeed. Responsibility for implementation of an effective profiling system will probably fall to the medical group administration.

Why Do Medical Groups Need Their Own Profiling System?

Physician practices are being profiled in many geographic regions for a number of purposes. Since provider profiles present information on physician practices, it should be clear that physicians and their group administrators should be intimately involved in the process and should be provided with the information that is of interest to physicians. The characteristics of a practice that should be reviewed by physician groups should provide insights that will allow physicians and their group practices to perform their health delivery role better and continue providing care on a financially sound basis. Historically, and with only a few exceptions, profiling endeavors have been undertaken by payers, with less-than-optimal provider involvement, and have been aimed at identifying providers who use more resources than others in treating their patients. Because these profiles are often not adjusted for case mix, this has usually meant that physicians or medical groups who treat patients with more significant problems are singled out as heavy users of services. The medical group that has attracted sicker patients will obviously have a tendency to use more resources per patient than other medical groups treating patients with less need for services. Therefore, profiling service use will be likely to show higher costs and have a tendency to penalize the groups with sicker patients. This has led many physicians to be concerned about their ability to continue to deliver appropriate care to their patients.

Providing feedback on how a physician or a medical group practice is providing care is a legitimate use for profiling, but physicians and medical groups should take the lead in ensuring that profiles are meaningful and fair to providers of care and ultimately to their patients. Profiling of physicians (or other providers, such as hospitals, health maintenance organizations, or integrated delivery networks) can fulfill this need if this work is done appropriately. The goal of physician profiling is to obtain a better understanding of the strengths and weaknesses of a medical practice. When physicians and their group practice administrators are responsible for deciding which parameters are profiled and how they are profiled, profiles will be relevant to them.

What Can Be Profiled?

Four questions are important in designing a profiling system:

- What is important to the physicians in the practice in order to make the physicians and patients better served?
- What information do others require about the practice? Physicians need to address the legitimate information needs of others as they design their systems.
- What is the practice already receiving from HMOs and insurance carriers in the way of reports?
- What is necessary to meet outstanding reporting needs? What data are necessary to meet those needs, and what resources are necessary to turn raw data into useful information?

The things that can be known about a practice and therefore profiled are essentially limitless in concept, but they are limited in reality because the necessary data are unavailable. The data immediately available to most practices are typically limited, and data limitations in turn will limit the immediate scope of profiling efforts.

New profiles can always be created, though there are some limitations. For example, in the normal course of business, simple financial profiles of the practice can be generated by comparing revenues to expenses or looking at costs categorized by procedure. Trends can be followed using relatively modest time and resources in addition to the time implied by external reporting requirements.

With a little extra effort, any practice can gather data from patients or other sources on a small number of important practice attributes. Targeted data can be relatively easily recorded for profiling purposes using personal computers. Without substantial effort, it is possible to record demographics and a small number of selected facts about patients, such as immunization history, patient compliance, or patient satisfaction. The scope of profiling must be contained if the goal is to use available resources. But even for a solo practice, knowing the trends in patient satisfaction or trends in patient compliance can be quite useful.

Finally, any data that are already computerized can often provide grist for profiling. When computers are used in the ordinary course of business to make appointments or record diagnoses and procedures in order to file claims or encounters, useful profiles can sometimes be generated with limited additional work. When extensive raw data must be taken from the patient record or from paper claim forms for profiling purposes alone, the cost of profiling these aspects may be high.

Don't Physicians Already Know How Their Practices Are Doing?

Few physicians know, from the ordinary course of their daily activities, how well their practices perform with respect to many relevant parameters. They certainly cannot know how their practices compare to others without a formal profiling effort. It is not likely that a physician will know the average number of visits delivered to patients with diabetes or the average length of stay for hospitalized patients unless someone else reports this information. Nor is it likely that the physician will know whether these statistics are attractive and whether a higher or lower number is to be desired. There was a time when analysts believed that a short average length of stay for a given mix of diagnosis-related groups was a good thing, but then someone discovered that a short length of stay could indicate that patients who were being admitted did not actually require hospital care. Similarly, a larger-than-average number of visits may be desirable if it reduces the need to hospitalize patients.

Interactions between physician and patient usually take place one at a time, extend over a long period, deal with multiple problems on multiple occasions, and lead to the full spectrum of outcomes. Therefore, physicians are not likely to know all they should about how their practice is faring unless they can consult a comparative profile. Measuring performance is complicated by the fact that, particularly for patients with serious problems, each physician is part of a team, and the outcome is the result of a team effort. Comparisons become even more difficult when several physicians with very different mixes of patients are profiled. Simplistic profiles generated without taking these factors into consideration have not been as useful as they could be.

To know how they are doing, physicians need systematic profiling based in part on data external to the practice. In short, they need a systematic means for keeping track of important practice activities and meaningful comparisons with the performance of peers, or an accepted standard, presented in an easy-to-read and useful format.

What Do Physicians Need to Know?

Physicians need to know whether there are better ways to treat patients, which referral providers are the best and give the most cost-effective care, and how their patients are doing. They need information that helps them to make better decisions in all areas of patient treatment they control. The state of the art of profiling does not yet provide the means to achieve this goal entirely, but that does not mean that we cannot select specific areas of importance to offer meaningful insights based on profiling data.

Outcomes and Patient Satisfaction

Physicians first need to know how best to treat their patients, what the outcomes of treatment are, and whether patients are satisfied with their care. If patients are happy with their care and are doing well, most physicians would believe that they are doing well. Physicians and their administrators also need to know whether patients are satisfied with the service they receive from nonmedical personnel and why (or why not). Measures of outcomes are more difficult to develop than measures of patient satisfaction, but neither is available without a systematic data gathering and profiling effort. (See Chapter Eight on patient satisfaction.)

Quality of Care

Quality can be defined as doing the right thing, in the right way, at the right time, the first time and every time. When quality of care is measured, implicitly or explicitly, it should be measured with this definition in mind.

Quality is often measured through protocol conformance, for example, rates of immunizations delivered to young children, Pap smears and mammography delivered to women in appropriate age groups, and eye exams for patients with diabetes (the right things at the right time), or through selected outcome information, such as infection rates, returns to operating room, death rates, and complication rates (the results of the wrong thing or the wrong time or the wrong way).

Quality cannot be strictly defined in terms of cost. Low cost can be an indicator of high quality, for example. Unnecessary procedures at a higher-than-necessary cost (not the right thing), multiple and expensive complications of treatment (not the right thing or not delivered in the right way), and untreated minor problems escalating to more serious and expensive problems (certainly not the right thing at the right time) increase costs but do not indicate high quality.

Financial Performance

In close conjunction with information on their patients' outcomes, satisfaction, and the quality of care delivered, physicians and administrators need to know how their practices are doing financially and how they will do in the future. If physicians do not cover their costs, they will go out of business and will stop caring for their patients. In the days of fee-for-service, financial performance was largely a question of volume, and trends in past financial performance alone could forecast the future. Prices and costs were always in the background, but most prices were set to cover costs. With managed care, capitation, bonuses, withholds, and shared risks, the equation is not so simple. Now that each physician's office, the lab, and the radiology department may be cost centers rather than pure profit centers, evaluating current and projecting future financial performance is complex. Physician groups are often at risk in one way or another for treatment delivered elsewhere, in hospitals or other physicians' offices. This means that they need to know in some detail about the performance of others in order to serve their patients and stay in business.

What Are the Limitations on Profiles?

Providing all information physicians need to know is usually not possible. All information has a cost, and the decision on which pieces of information can be provided is typically based on interactions among the state of the art, cost, and the value of the information to be provided. In some instances, the cost of analysis is low and data already exist in a usable form. In other cases, however, the costs of acquiring, analyzing, and reporting new raw data may be too high. Usually the data already available to most physician practices do not support all profiling endeavors. From the standpoint of the physician or group practice, the primary limitation on generating new profiles is the availability of relatively reliable raw data. Some practices have requested and received data on their patients from their HMOs; these comprehensive data allow for construction of comprehensive episodes of care or population-based analyses.

Much of the information necessary to profile outcomes, satisfaction, costs, or the quality of care delivered by a practice is unavailable because it has never been gathered or is in someone else's possession. This applies to data specific to the patients served by a practice and to data necessary to provide comparisons in the local market.

Even in the context of a physician's role as a strict gatekeeper in an HMO where all services provided must be approved by the primary care physician (PCP), physicians usually know very little about what happens to their patients once they leave the office unless the HMO tells them. Even in fully computerized physicians' offices, the physician may have access only to information on what was approved, not on what was actually delivered or how much it cost. Unless an HMO provides access to the complete patient claims record, information will be limited to services delivered directly by the practice, what has been ordered by the practice, what has been authorized by the practice, or data that have been independently gathered by the practice. Services actually delivered by others will usually remain a mystery unless those others provide the data. The PCP and the practice probably have even less access to information on services delivered by other providers outside the practice to patients covered by plans that are less restrictive with respect to authorization of services. If outside services can be obtained by patients without PCP approval, the practice will not even have a record of the authorization.

Without the relatively comprehensive data available from health plans, a physician cannot easily get a complete and accurate picture of the delivered patient services. Moreover, without relatively complete data, the produced information can be difficult to interpret. The totals, averages, ratios, and rates that make up most service delivery analyses cannot be accurately calculated with incomplete data. Practices should request as much external data as they can, and they may increase their internal data gathering. Most practices should expand data available, but there are clearly many questions that the practice can answer with available data, and those should be answered first.

Thus, the first and most important restriction on the production of profiles is the availability of relatively complete data on patients served by a practice with reference to the questions being asked. The second is the availability of comparable data on comparable patients served by other practices. And the third is the availability of personnel and tools that allow for the production of meaningful reports that can summarize the data covering patients served and comparable services provided to other patients.

Can an Accurate Picture of Practice Patterns Be Found Without Comprehensive Data?

The straightforward answer to this question is no. This does not mean that very important insights into practice patterns cannot be gained with incomplete data, but it is necessary to recognize that more comprehensive data allow more comprehensive analyses. Three examples illustrate this point.

• Incomplete data suffice in instances where they are not incomplete with reference to the question. A practice seeking to know how many imaging procedures its patients receive in the process of treating fractures typically requires other people's data. Alternatively, a practice wishing to know how many imaging procedures it delivers to patients with fractures can usually answer this question. In other words, by asking a more specific question, clinics are likely to have the capability to glean meaningful information.

• Relatively complete data can be gathered when necessary to answer some questions. Most pediatric practices strive to ensure that their patients are receiving appropriate immunizations, and in the ordinary course of business, many gather data on the immunizations delivered by the practice in a computer system. These data can often be summarized relatively easily. But it is unlikely that any organization has complete records on patients seen by a practice regarding immunizations. Children seen by the practice may have received their immunizations from other sources, like public health clinics or other pediatricians outside the practice, and sometimes parents have failed to obtain scheduled immunizations for their children in spite of the best efforts of the pediatrician. Therefore, if pediatricians wish to know about their patients' immunization records and the reasons for recording an incomplete course of immunizations, the practice must gather some of the information from parents or from records that others provide. The physician practice is the best potential source of summary information on this topic since it provides services and has access to parents and patients.

• There is a need to get data from other sources. If the practice determines that the total cost of care provided to the patients served by the practice is of interest, rather than just information on care provided by the practice, it is not likely that this information can be obtained from any source other than the carrier. Even a reasonable approximation of the truth is unlikely to be discovered by a professional practice without external cooperation. As a compounding complication, patient confidentiality issues may preclude the sharing of patient-specific information. Without information on services delivered by other providers of health care services, the limitation, if severe enough, may absolutely preclude meaningful analysis of some important questions.

How Do We Profile Specialists?

The simple answer is "with great difficulty." Different specialists face a differing mix of morbidity requiring different approaches and yielding different outcomes. In addition, they find themselves to be part of a team, and different members of the team provide different services driven by timing of need and availability. For example, a rural cardiologist is likely to have more visits per patient, holding morbidity constant, because there is no partner or cardiologist across the hall to cover and share the load. There are differences in the patients referred as well; the cardiologist in a fee-for-service, self-referred environment is likely to see different patients from one in a gatekeeper model. And a cardiologist at a regional medical school in a gatekeeper model is likely to see even a different set of patients.

The approaches to solving these problems of data availability and analysis usually involve some form of case mix adjustment and analysis of episodes of care. The source of data is usually the medical claim, and even if it were supplemented with extensive other information, these are clouded by definitional entries; there is seldom a claim for cardiac bypass surgery that does not indicate the appropriate level of occlusion or other appropriate diagnosis on the claim. Benchmark data are often difficult to obtain, and even when available, their applicability to an individual specialty practice is questionable. Further, providers that do surgery when it is not necessary often look better on an episode basis, with lower death rates, fewer complications, fewer returns to the operating room, fewer readmits, and a lower cost per case simply because their patients are healthier and it is difficult to do comprehensive case mix adjustment. We all expect the cardiac surgeon specializing in emergency bypasses to look worse on an episode basis than one who performs surgery on marginal cases where the need is equivocal. In some cases we can adjust for this difficulty; in most cases we cannot.

To help avoiding misinterpretation, there are a few general rules that can be applied. One of these is that any system that analyzes services delivered by an individual specialist without regard to those delivered by others will give incomplete and possibly very misleading information. Another is that analyses based on episodes of care alone will reward the provider doing marginally unnecessary or completely unnecessary procedures if the analysis is procedure based, as it often is for many specialties. Specialists should be profiled based on what happens to the patients they see and on population parameters in addition to episodes they are assigned and the work they perform. An individual medical group will usually have difficulty performing these analyses, even with appropriate benchmarks, because the number of patients is too small. A health plan has a better opportunity of doing these analyses, but results must be viewed very carefully to be sure that the analysis does not punish the best and reward the marginal.

How Do Practices Find Comparable Data?

In order to provide analyses of a practice that have a meaning for a given period, it is necessary to have relevant comparisons, norms, or benchmarks. Practices can usually ascertain improvement or deterioration in selected practice pattern attributes over time without external benchmarks or standards, but external measures are critical for a single period or if the goal is to see how a practice ranks when compared to other practices. Even when there are well-established protocols or standards of practice, these are seldom achieved; how close is good enough requires comparisons. When standards are not available, the experience of other practices must be used for comparison. For some purposes, the local experience of other providers—that is, local norms—will be most meaningful. For others, national norms will be appropriate for comparison, and for still others, best-practice norms will be most appropriate. Sometimes all three of these normative comparisons are useful.

Benchmarks are sometimes available for measures such as visits per member, discharges per thousand, average length of stay, and procedures per thousand for most of the common procedures. These are provided by consulting firms, commercial data repositories, public agencies, and a number of industry and professional associations, such as the Center for Research in Ambulatory Health Care Administration. Since practices differ in the types of patients they serve, however, these norms may need adjustment to be meaningful. Available benchmarks can be misleading if they were not developed for a specific type of practice, and they can be very misleading if a practice is relying on data that are more or less incomplete than the data that generated the benchmark. In general, any substantial differences between data used to profile a practice and the data used to generate benchmarks must be taken into consideration, or the benchmarks will not be applicable. Substantial differences can include any differences in composition of the data used, differences in age and sex distribution, geographic differences (particularly those driven by patient expectations), benefit plan differences, the specific relative value scale used, provider specialty, mix of diagnoses treated and comorbidities, range of services offered by a provider, and, if costs are used in any way, local price structures.

Who Should Be Involved in Implementing a New Profiling Effort?

In the best of all possible worlds, everyone with a need for information and everyone affected by a profiling system should participate in defining and implementing the effort. This is unlikely to happen, however, especially in small professional practices.

Small practices often find it difficult to field the effort. Larger practices know that limitations on data availability, comparative data, and other factors will make some categories of results difficult to obtain. Even fielding an effort to make sense of profiles already being received can be very difficult for hard-pressed practice managers seeking to know what can be gained before expending resources.

In spite of these difficulties, every practice should make an effort to report on critical success factors, and profiling offers this opportunity. Even a limited effort formalizes the process to some degree and begins the process of using the information gathered as a regular part of the management process. If the practice can afford the effort, the more thorough the involvement is, the better the result will be.

Those in the practice who seek information and know what information should be useful must take the lead. In some practices, the practicing physicians will be the prime movers; in others, practice managers must show the way. But in any case, it is critical that the first efforts bear some fruit if the ultimate goal of providing useful information to decision makers is to be reached.

The list of those who should participate differs from practice to practice. Sometimes a single individual will be designed to select reporting methodologies and set implementation priorities in addition to technical staff. A comprehensive process would include individual physicians, medical directors, chief financial officer, chief information officer, nursing director, staff nurses, laboratory director, chief radiology technician, manager of information systems, analysts, and others with interests, including those who manage the appointment-making process and legal risk management. It would also be useful to involve representatives from important HMOs and other providers; indeed, outside consulting assistance may make the difference between success and failure. While this list is daunting, a single individual with the right knowledge and skills can begin the process.

What Approaches to Profiling Implementation Are Available?

There are essentially five approaches to the implementation of profiling: build-it-yourself; buy a ready-made package, which usually involves some substantial customized consulting; hire a consultant to build and implement it; use a service bureau; or arrange for another organization already doing profiling to do the analysis to your specifications. The actual implementation may be a combination of these approaches.

Build It Yourself

This option is immediately appealing to many. Practices with practice management computer systems usually have some built-in reporting capability, which can provide any set of useful information supported by the data in the system. For self-generated data, this may be more than adequate, especially if the system has been in place for an extended period and reporting on trends can be implemented. Benchmarks are probably not built into the system, but internal comparisons may suffice initially. Nevertheless, in almost every instance, there are major pieces of information that cannot be developed without external data.

Among the advantages of building it yourself are the development of customized reporting, control of the analytic approach, and apparently low cost. The disadvantages usually involve time considerations, since internal staff usually already have full-time jobs, difficulty in implementing some of the complex algorithms necessary, lack of comprehensiveness, and lack of sufficient internal expertise. Unless the profiling goal is only a few simple reports that require no external benchmarks and little data external to the practice management system, build-it-yourself profiling implementation is not likely to provide a viable solution except for extremely large practices.

Buy a Ready-Made Package

This approach is appealing since it seems to offer a quick and easy way to implement a profiling effort. If the practice seeks a comprehensive and relatively immediate solution, purchase of a ready-made system will be the option of choice, especially when the product comes with substantial customized consulting effort. Those who develop packages have applied significant effort to incorporate tools, techniques, and algorithms that make the information generated potentially more valuable. On the other hand, at least some of these built-in capabilities can be difficult to implement in specific practices due to data limitations and specific local conditions; other expensive system attributes may be irrelevant to a specific practice. This approach is usually quicker and more comprehensive but less targeted and can be more or less expensive than other alternatives with more or less return. Most ready-made products must be highly customized in order to meet the needs of most medical groups, and there is no ready-made solution to all problems.

Hire a Consultant and Build a Customized Package

This approach can provide precisely what the practice needs and derive information from the available data without an underlying ready-made package. A customized approach usually requires longer lead times and higher cost for a more limited product. But if the practice needs are well defined and relatively limited, this can be by far the best solution since the client can get precisely what is desired and does not pay for unneeded capabilities.

Use a Service Bureau

A service bureau (send it the data and it will prepare the profiles) is often in the background when a ready-made product is licensed. In fact, service bureaus often use a ready-made product to generate profiling reports.

This option may be only a slight modification on the other approaches. The practice usually does not avoid all the work in implementing a system in-house since data must be extracted and provided to the service bureau and reports must be evaluated for reasonableness before they are distributed. Because those who offer services of this type specialize in this activity, they have highly specialized staffs and extensive experience with data idiosyncrasies. Under the right circumstances, this approach can provide targeted reporting at less cost than internal reporting.

Arrange for Another Organization to Do the Analysis

This approach offers several potential advantages and some clear disadvantages. An HMO or an integrated delivery network usually has much more comprehensive data than are available to any individual practice. The effort it has put into creating profiles can be applied to many practices, providing them with economies of scale. This may be the best and only approach available to most practices if local benchmarks are to be obtained. If reports received are combined internally and supplemented with internal reporting, particularly using internal data that are not available to the overarching organization, a viable result may be attained.

The biggest disadvantage of this approach is that the concerns of others may continue to determine what is reported, and reporting will be segmented and not comparable if multiple carriers or other sources are involved. Most practices will get externally generated profiles whether they request them or not, so efforts applied to getting external organizations to modify profiles to suit a practice's specific needs may also make these externally generated profiles more useful, and they are certainly inexpensive.

How Much Time and Effort Does Profiling Require?

The amount of time, resources, and effort involved in implementing a profiling system is largely determined by the goals of the system, the approach, and whether extensive external data gathering and comprehensive reporting on all activities of practitioners in the practice are involved. Simple profiles generated from available internal data can be designed and generated using a fraction of a full-time employee; extensive external data gathering and extensive analysis can require a department of several employees supplemented with commercial software licenses and substantial external consulting. The amount of resources required is a direct function of the nature of the effort.

If the goal is to implement a comprehensive profiling system using external and internal data, accomplishing the task can be expensive in terms of the time and effort of existing staff, new staff, equipment, software, and external consultants. Extensive time is required for planning, reviewing alternatives, getting approvals, acquiring and evaluating data, implementing or designing and modifying software, and educating the audience, and continuing modification may require significant part-time commitments from many in the organization, as well as substantial expenditure on outside experts in both the implementation and continued maintenance phases. The cost can be high, but the rewards can be substantial.

Conclusion

The quantity and type of information that will be necessary to operate successfully in future modes of medical service delivery require a substantial commitment of time and effort. Practice profiling was once an anomaly and not a concern. Now everyone is either producing profiles, receiving profiles, or about to do so. Some of these profiles are of use to the medical group practice; some are not.

Making profiling information more useful will provide opportunities for physicians to improve the performance of their practices in terms of quality of care, patient satisfaction, and financial performance. In the process of determining how to lay the appropriate foundation for a practice-based profiling effort, the potential impact of the new information on internal performance or on external perception must be ascertained first. The practice needs to understand why profiling is important in the light of its goals and objectives, and providers need to be intimately involved in the process if maximum gains are to be achieved. Planning, obtaining data, and implementing and maintaining a profiling system can provide substantial rewards if it is done appropriately.

CHAPTER TWO

WHAT DATA ARE NEEDED FOR PHYSICIAN PROFILES?

Manon Spitzer Ruben, Peter Braun, Philip Caper

Data are a fundamental determinant of successful physician profiles. Yet identification of data sources and selection of data elements and enhancement tools are not the first requirements of health care administrators developing this activity. Rather, the first and most important decision is seeking and achieving consensus on profiling objectives. The second is establishing criteria for and identifying providers to be profiled, which includes examining characteristics of the specialty, financial relationships, or practice settings that influence profile design, data requirements, and the choice of analytic methods. The intended audiences for profiles should be identified during the articulation of profiling objectives, and their needs must be clearly understood in terms of communication style, the media for delivery of information, and resources to support the dialogue around the profiling process. An organization will be well served by investing resources in developing consensus not only on major objectives, but also on criteria for who and what is to be measured, how it is to be measured and reported, how the results will be used, and how the overall effort will be evaluated.

Objective Setting and Data

A health plan, provider group, or other health care entity may embark on physician profile development for many reasons. Clear identification and prioritization of objectives is imperative to inform the selection of data, determine the analytic dimensions, and assess the scale and expense of resources for development, production, and support of the profiling effort. Successful profiles create desired incentives and change behavior in measurable ways.

Health plans or other health care entities can launch the effort to locate, evaluate, assemble, and document source data for profiles parallel to the administrative and managerial activities around articulation of profiling objectives. A sober assessment of the availability, scope, quality, and timeliness of data that are central to even the most basic profiling efforts should inform all other decisions. Any strategies that promise "one size fits all" should be viewed with some skepticism. Limitations will become quickly apparent when discussions proceed regarding objectives, the profile subjects, and the mode of analysis, in part because the profile concept seeks to focus attention by being short and succinct. Physician profiles developed in support of medical management and quality improvement objectives, for example, emphasize clinical data presented in terms of process and outcome measures for member and patient populations. Profiles oriented toward resource efficiency, cost reduction, or improved profitability typically focus on the financial dimensions of physician decisions about resources invested in patient care. Profiles that meet requirements for accreditation, like the Health Plan Employer and Data Information Set (HEDIS), or seek to reinforce employer group satisfaction and member retention imply still different criteria for data selection, measurement tools, and reporting style.

Core Data

Most source data for profiles currently derive from billing claims and encounter records, enrollment and eligibility systems, and ad hoc reference systems describing physician specialty and geographic location, financial relationships, and practice group affiliation. Data requirements depend on the type of profiling report a practice wishes to generate. Certain data will be part of most reports: a unique patient identification, member date of birth, member sex, ICD–9 (International Classification of Disease, Ninth Revision, Clinical Modification) codes, and claim numbers. For inpatient provider profiles, fields for admit and discharge dates and length of stay, and discharge status are of interest. An outpatient profile might include the date of service or maybe an emergency room flag. Other data fields to consider are X-ray data, referral information, and pharmacy fields. For pharmacy profiles, prescribing physician or physician specialist and filling provider should be added to the profiling database. Although there is accelerating development of electronic media to record clinical experience at the point of service, these are generally still confined to a minority of medical groups and are not yet available with sufficient uniformity or scope to support profiling efforts. (Evidence-based profiling reports are discussed in Chapter Four.)

Each of the conventional legacy systems for processing and capturing data was created to serve a specific function in the organization, not for provider profiling activity. As a consequence, the data they capture and store, which may function validly for their original purpose, must be evaluated from different perspectives for provider profiles. Ironically, health plans, especially large and well-established plans, generally experience their greatest difficulty in assembling accurate, systematic information about their providers from the ad hoc sources. Common problems are multiple provider identification numbers; unknown, inaccurate, or dual-specialty-type designations; multiple practice locations; unknown practice group affiliation; and nonsystematic information on financial relationships for each product. Each of these different problems means that the profile design managers must explore the scope of issues raised, develop decision criteria, and apply them to the raw data before such information can be used as data elements for end user profiles.

Demographic Data from Enrollment and Eligibility Systems

Conventional eligibility and enrollment data sources offer important information for planning profiles. The first category is data on the demographic characteristics not only of patients but also on all members who are eligible to receive services. Both are needed because managed care profiling objectives require population-based as well as patient-based statistical approaches. Depending on the organizational setting, a population-based analysis could include demographic data on all members of a managed care plan, all indemnity subscribers and their dependents, all Medicaid recipients, Medicare beneficiaries, and so on. Only population-based analysis allows identification of access barriers or failures, for whatever reason, to reach all relevant populations with preventive services such as mammography, colorectal cancer screening, influenza vaccinations, prenatal care, and well-child immunizations. On the other hand, exploration of the practice patterns of referral specialists such as endocrinologists and cardiothoracic surgeons can be confined to evidence from the claims and enrollment systems on each physician's own patients.

No profiling effort can proceed without, at a minimum, a data element that uniquely identifies each eligible member or patient, the age and gender of the individual, and dates enrolled or disenrolled. This requirement seems simple enough on the surface, but with data, the devil is always in the details. For example, some organizations have to invest resources to create a unique eligible identification for spouses and dependents because the enrollment system, designed for tracking premiums, records information on only the contract holder and on the policy type (two-person, family). Similarly plans often fail to create an independent record for a newborn at the time of delivery and do so only after several months. As a consequence, billing claims submitted by pediatricians sometimes literally indicate that well-child services and childhood inoculations were delivered to the mothers. The way that age is recorded in the enrollment file (date of birth is best) determines whether age in combination with a claim or encounter record can be calculated appropriately to produce accurate primary care physician profiles that evaluate performance relative to measures required by HEDIS. Finally, the way that eligibility is recorded (start and end dates) and the frequency with which eligibility status is confirmed can be stumbling blocks for profiling approaches that differentiate process measures or outcomes based on continuous enrollment.

Enrollment and eligibility systems can supply a wealth of additional data to support development of more sophisticated provider profiles. For example, these files should include data identifying an eligible member's zip code of residence, employer, health plan and product, benefit type and coverage codes, and primary care physician (PCP) assignment (along with dates of enrollment or disenrollment if PCP assignment changes). If the enrollee or patient is a Medicaid recipient or Medicare beneficiary, eligibility classification and disability status are highly desirable data elements.

Information derived from sources extraneous to claims or conventional eligibility sources can also be incorporated into this environment and made relevant to the subsequent physician profiles. A health plan might have administered postenrollment risk assessment, functional status, or member satisfaction questionnaires to all Medicare beneficiaries, for example. It could record the scores as an enhancement to ordinary enrollment information and make the data available to primary care providers and administrative coordinators. Similarly, plans can flag the enrollment record to designate patients as outliers relative to stop-loss reinsurance or other plan-specified thresholds. In order for this type of outlier information to be used appropriately in a provider profile, it must always be recorded with the enrollment information of the member or patient, because the status can never be determined from a single claim or from a single provider's experience.

Claim and Encounter Data

Claim and encounter data supply the bulk of information used in all types of provider profiles. This is the source of information that tells whether a medical event occurred and for what reason (diagnosis), what service or services were delivered by which providers at what sites, and usually some quantification of economic value. Ideally a health plan or other health care entity will have access to data for all types of service and providers for all their members or patients: inpatient records in the form of a single confinement summary (admission to discharge) or in day-to-day detail; facility outpatient records in line item detail; all records for care in any other facility; and all data on ambulatory services, laboratory tests, and prescriptions from all providers in all settings.

If these data are to be integrated in a repository such as a data warehouse or datamart to support profiling (which is highly recommended), the data model must take into account that these records will represent every clinical and financial classification system used in the health care industry. These will generally include ICD–9 diagnosis and procedure codes, diagnosis-related group (DRG), CPTs (physician's current procedural terminology) and HCPCS (the Health Care Financing Administration's common procedure coding system), and, the bane of all analysis, local codes, which must be identified and documented. The minefields represented here cannot be overstated. One client recently had to restart a physician profile effort after three months when it discovered that in the context of a uniform "facility" claim layout, it had used a field that was designated CPT code, unused for the inpatient records, to record a local administrative code indicating a hospital's payment status. The software system that logically groups individual claims to create treatment episodes across delivery sites quite properly interpreted the entries as CPT codes, contaminating the accuracy of all episodes involving hospitalization.

Clinical and Service Code Data

The number and specificity of ICD–9 diagnosis and procedure codes as well as the specificity of CPT codes is vitally important to successful profiles, regardless of objectives. These not only support clinically focused quality objectives and financially focused business objectives but also enable the use of new software systems for risk assessment. These health risk assessments facilitate both enhancement programs such as disease management and adjustment of capitation or other financial arrangements. More data are always better data. Only ICD–9 diagnosis codes taken to a fourth or sometimes fifth digit can distinguish important acuity levels. For example, clients often record only the three-digit ICD–9 code for diabetes mellitus (250), whereas the decimal extensions distinguish among patients who have diabetes mellitus without complication (250.0), life-threatening ketoacidosis (250.1), and hyperosmolar coma (250.2), each with different implications for resource use. ICD–9 procedure codes at the fourth and fifth digits distinguish between, for example, heart surgery patients who undergo single coronary artery bypass grafts from those receiving quadruple coronary artery bypass grafts. The CPT modifiers, among other things, place a physician's role in an event in perspective, distinguishing between principal and assistant surgeons. Failure to recognize and accommodate these distinctions can seriously jeopardize the results, leading analysts to overstate the true rate of certain procedures and understate their true costs.

Depending on the organizational perspective from which profiling is undertaken, there is no guarantee of consistency in the way that the ICD–9 and CPT codes appear in the claim and encounter data files. Indeed there is a high probability of inconsistency in the initial data capture. A health plan must scrutinize data from thousands of providers. If a large multispecialty medical group seeks to profile its physicians, it may need to transform data to achieve consistency if it has been complying with different health plan reporting requirements, as well as Medicaid and Medicare reporting formats.

Financial Data

The most troublesome issue for profiles that include any economic measures—and all profiles should have some economic content—is the inconsistency of financial information. If a provider is rendering services to patients under a full or partial capitation arrangement, records of each encounter often contain no entries for what under fee-for-service claims would be charged, allowed, and paid amounts. Alternatively they may contain a proxy allowed amount from a fee schedule that represents the financial liability that would have been incurred. Moreover, with exceptions such as Kaiser Permanente, almost no providers operate for all patients under a genuinely global capitation; some services and some patients always remain outside the capitation scope. Data for commercial managed care health maintenance organizations (HMOs) and for large multispecialty provider groups are typically a mixture, with some services included in the capitation amounts and others discounted fee-for-service.

Actual allowed dollars also vary depending on the deals that each hospital or medical group negotiates with commercial payers and managed care plans, and to a lesser degree even in Medicaid and Medicare, because of adjustments for teaching status or disproportionate share provider status. Paid amounts are the most variable and difficult to document and interpret if the physicians are serving patients from more than one payer source, and even within one payer source if it offers multiple products. Paid amounts vary depending on the insurance product, the benefit type and coverage, and patient copayments and deductibles, in addition to variation in negotiated rates by hospital, medical group, and geographic location. In the end, all data represented by dollars are accurate only insofar as the context for their interpretation is known.

The degree of difficulty in contending with these issues varies with the nature of the health care entity that is assembling and developing data for physician profiling and the number of different data sources they must understand and interpret relative to each physician or group. Increasingly, analysts dealing with professional data use relative value units (RVUs) in parallel with other financial data to help normalize their measures of resource value, whether or not they use the Resource-Based Relative-Value Scale (RBRVS) as part of their payment strategy.[1] Similar options exist for normalizing facility inpatient data, for fixing each DRG value according to Medicare values or similar formula, and for hospital outpatient facilities.

A far more troublesome data issue in a capitated or mixed reimbursement environment is the difficulty of estimating the extent of nonreporting of service events and the associated details on diagnosis and treatment when providers have no financial incentive to report. Our experience has demonstrated that in the absence of enforceable penalties, reporting of encounter data is highly variable among physicians and between groups and, in managed Medicaid and Medicare, among participating health plans. As a consequence, apparent variation among physicians in rates of office visits and for preventive care services is so extreme that a profile effort can immediately lose credibility except as evidence of inconsistent reporting compliance.

Claim and encounter data also typically carry information establishing the place of service and facility identifier, type of service, and date of service. Along with the data on clinical diagnoses and procedures, data like these can extend the spectrum of profiling beyond simple audit-style descriptions of provider activities toward valuable refinements such as risk assessment (morbidity or severity) and adjustment. Whether and how these enhancements are pursued depends on business objectives, the type of providers profiled, the nature and sophistication of the intended audience, and presentation medium and support.

Profile Focus: Physicians and Other Providers

The scope of data required to support physician profiling and the way data are organized and treated analytically vary substantially depending on the type of provider, the providers' relationship to members and patients, and the analytic tools deemed appropriate for achieving the desired business objectives. These will also differ depending on the nature of the entity undertaking the profile activity. For the purposes of this examination, we assume the perspective of an insurance plan, which may be a managed care organization, a multiproduct Blue Cross and Blue Shield, or a provider-sponsored organization (PSO) functioning as a risk-bearing entity.

Physicians and other providers may be addressed in profiles as individual practitioners within a specialty or as interacting participants within practice groups or clinics. If the units for comparative analysis are groups, these may be single-specialty or multispecialty groups. Primary care specialists such as family practice, internal medicine, and pediatrics are often members of multispecialty groups, and occasionally joined under the same administrative umbrella by specialists in obstetrics and gynecology. On the other hand, single-specialty groups are more common for referral care. A cardiology practice often consists of several evaluation and management specialists, one or more cardiologists who concentrate on diagnostic imaging and other testing procedures, those who perform balloon angioplasty but no invasive surgical procedures, and perhaps a couple of cardiac surgeons for valve and coronary artery bypass operations. Each of these configurations presents a challenge for data availability, selection, and analytic treatment. Data from the ad hoc systems on provider attributes can be immensely valuable for establishing genuine peer groups for comparative analysis, which is central to the profiling concept. Otherwise development of credible profiles is inevitably an iterative process whose first phase serves essentially only to facilitate identification of apples and oranges.

Another fundamental distinction for profiling purposes is between physicians who are accountable for an assigned panel of members and are financially at risk for all or substantial portions of members' care for all types of services (PCPs), and those who are accountable only for the patients to whom they deliver care.

PCP Profiles

The best PCP profiles consist of two parts. The first requires data on all the assigned members, including those who have not had any service during the profiling period, and data from claim and encounter systems from all providers for all types of care. This phase of the profile should include a summary of members' demographic characteristics, ideally including a measure of morbidity as well as age and gender. Data should be assembled to report on the percentage of members who had no claim and on the average length of eligibility and rate of turnover among the assigned panel. Utilization data can be misleading for a physician whose members are all recent enrollees compared to one whose panel has well-established relationships because the calculations of rates of service are based on services per member per year or per month. If the PCP status is recent and enrollment is growing rapidly, an annualized member year for any specific age and gender segment will concatenate experiences for several individuals. The resulting pattern of service may look very different from a rate for members who are continuously eligible through the same time period.

A comprehensive PCP profile also presents summary utilization and financial information on the members' rates of use of hospital inpatient and outpatient resources, primary care and referred medical and surgical services, and, if available, prescription drug and other resources. These may be complemented by selected utilization and cost highlights, perhaps representing an organization's consensus on key improvements, such as reducing emergency department visits and increasing rates for preventive care services. This part of the profile serves as an assessment of the PCP's care coordinator function for members' total resource consumption and for delivery system performance.

The second part of the profile consists of an examination of each PCP's direct contribution to the members' overall resource consumption and uses data only from the PCP's own claim or encounter records. It looks at what specific services this PCP delivered to his or her patients and what percentage of the overall member panel's needs the PCP met. Here, an organization will need to decide how to aggregate individual CPT codes, or CPT codes in combination with ICD–9 diagnosis codes, into medically meaningful units that communicate a picture of the care experience of patients. This type of profile allows an organization to evaluate performance against expectations at a number of different points, such as whether a PCP appears to supply 50 percent or 90 percent of the panel's ambulatory care or whether every asthmatic child is always referred to specialists.

Physician Specialist Profiles

Any physician not acting as a PCP relative to a set of members may be considered a specialist for the purposes of this chapter. Comparative profiles of individuals and practice groups must be developed within the context of a peer group for each specialty. Sometimes it is also necessary to differentiate by subspecialty. This will usually involve extensive examination of the service data represented in claim and encounter systems, and sometimes enrollment files as well, and consensus on criteria for grouping physicians into one class or another. Among physicians who record their specialty as cardiologist, for example, there is typically a broad spectrum of actual service mix. Do you consider the cardiologists who perform fewer than five diagnostic catheterizations per year representing 8 percent of their allowed dollars as members of the same peer group as cardiologists who perform seventy-five or more caths per year representing 65 percent of their allowed dollars?

Internal medicine doctors present a different and more subtle challenge. In fact, in terms of the CPT codes represented in the service mix, there is little to distinguish internal medicine from family practice or general practice. Where differences exist, they are more subtle and are related to the type of patient treated, the spectrum of diagnoses addressed without referring to another type of physician, and what might be called treatment or management intensity. Another matter is subspecialization. Judged only by the data describing their interactions with patients available to analysts in the form of ICD–9 diagnosis codes and CPT service codes, there is often little to differentiate an internal medicine specialist from some cardiologists and pulmonologists. Indeed, the lines must be drawn not around data but based on a plan or provider group's expectations of how each physician is to function in the environment.

Most health care plans concentrate the bulk of their profiling efforts around primary care specialists, including those who function as PCPs, and referral medical specialists such as gastroenterologists and cardiologists rather than surgeons. There are two principal reasons for this, and both involve data. First, administrative data sources typically lack the type of clinical content or precision—information, for example, on cancer stage or the degree of arterial occlusion—required to make an intelligent evaluation of the appropriateness of the surgery, the type of surgery performed, its cost, or its outcome. Second, although surgeons are accountable for their actions during and immediately pre- and postsurgery, they are typically engaged in a patient's care only on a transient basis and on referral from an evaluation and management specialist. Although administrative data may allow one to document a passage of time from the moment a diagnosis leading to surgery was first recorded, it gives only indirect evidence of the criteria for decision making leading to a recommendation for a surgical referral. As a consequence, profiles of surgical specialists tend either to emphasize descriptive attributes, such as service mix and cost, or are components of patient-centered episode analysis.

The Pursuit of Perfect Data

The caveats already stated regarding ICD–9 and CPT data and coding practices require even more serious attention when they are used to profile specialists. First, the narrower the specialty is, the fewer service and diagnosis codes are represented in the claim and encounter data sources, and thus there is a greater need for precision for any differentiation to occur. Second, case-mix adjustment software such as Adjusted Clinical Groups (ACGs) and Diagnosis Cost Groups (DCGs),[2] described in Chapter Five, rely on diagnosis codes to create hierarchies by acuity and comorbidity. These codes are also used for concurrent and prospective prediction by identifying those medical conditions that are most likely associated with continuing or accelerating high costs.

Caveats regarding all data for charged, allowed, or paid dollars are especially relevant for any specialist profiling activity. Although only a small minority of specialists are in capitated contracts, variation in the amounts charged is extreme and, excepting Medicare's RBRVS payment system, allowed and paid amounts may be equally variable depending on the payer, insurance product, and financial relationship. Clients are well advised to conduct their evaluations of the economic impact of differing practice patterns and case mix by adopting a parallel fixed and consistent system to quantify units of value such as RVUs.

No organization has perfect data, and no vendor's analytic tool set can protect clients from every misstep and minefield. The greatest danger is in doing nothing, for no one ever invests in improving data unless the cost of not doing so is not only obvious but sometimes even painful. On the positive side, few data sources are so abysmally bad that nothing of value can be developed.

Analytic Dimensions of Provider Profiles

The first step in developing the analytic dimensions of health care provider profiling is a set of decisions about what to measure and how the measures are to be applied and presented. Ideally, statistical measures are presented in a comparative framework and address multiple data points from the perspectives of patients, physicians or other providers, and administrative management.

Resource and Episode Perspectives

The first decision is selecting the units of analysis. The simplest profiling approaches use purely descriptive presentations of data on utilization and cost of resources represented by CPT service codes, recording the volume of occurrences, the number of patients, average dollars per service (charged, allowed, and paid), and aggregate dollars for each service and for the provider overall. The only virtue of these approaches is simplicity. More commonly, CPT codes are aggregated and sometimes qualified by combination with specific diagnosis codes to form more medically relevant treatment resource units. These are presented as rates per thousand members or patients and compared to benchmark rates within a plan or to external standards, with or without adjustment for differences in age and gender composition. Still more sophisticated profiles adjust also for member and patient morbidity to address the challenge that "my patients are sicker" (and thus more costly).

Data on services, diagnoses, and costs can also be aggregated to episodes of care for specific medical conditions, and these can be adjusted for age and gender and for morbidity. Episode analysis, if based on the most commonly used grouper software in current use, Episode Treatment Groups from Symmetry Health Data Systems, requires assembly of all data from claim and encounter systems from all types of providers and sites of service for a two-year period. Use of data on eligibility is optional. All the data caveats apply, and with even greater emphasis on assessment of the quality of each data source for profiling objectives before grouping to episodes. Deficiencies and inaccuracies in data for specific elements or from specific providers or sites may go undetected or will be more difficult to disentangle once the episode has been created.

Both the resource perspective and the episode approach have merits. For complex episodes, several providers typically contribute over time to the course of care for an individual patient. Although it is possible to identify each provider's contributions, usually an episode is assigned only to the physician who initiates the care. Analysts who wish to characterize the totality of a provider's performance relative to all his or her patients develop a resource view parallel to the episode perspective.

Audience for Profiles, Communication Style, and Medium

The most common audience for provider profile data is providers. Our experience indicates that the best results are obtained when profiling data are initially used only internally, sharing among medical directors and others involved in administration and medical management. Once field-tested on this limited scale, they can be disseminated to all providers who are participating in a health plan, medical group, or other business entity. It is imperative to document the planning process and objectives, as well as sources for and treatment of all the data, as well as any applications, for example, of risk assessment methods. Every measure, the data from which it derives, and how it is constructed should be described and illustrated, particularly with reference to the selection of benchmark standards for comparative information.

Everyone who undertakes a provider profiling activity must resolve the dilemma of communicating enough information and sufficient data to be meaningful without communicating too much data with too much complexity to be understood or acted on. There is no formula. In general, the more distant the intended audience is from the events that generate the data and the systems that record them, the greater the communication challenge and need for simplicity. At the same time, they cannot be so simplified that they will not achieve the objectives of providing incentives for changing behavior, regardless of focus. The most successful profiling efforts have been those in which health plan medical directors prepare the profile subjects and audience in advance with examples of the types of data and measures they will receive.

Data for profiles intended for employers or the general public usually provide aggregate measures of provider and plan performance rather than individual physician data. Although there have been sporadic attempts in California and New York to provide report cards on providers, these have been focused largely on hospital-based procedures, such as heart bypass operations and other procedures that have more dramatic potential than day-to-day medical practice. No consensus exists concerning what the public wants to know about providers and how the information should be communicated.

Most provider profiles to date are delivered in print media, supplemented by on-site presentations involving administration and provider representatives. However, the ability to "drill down" into the numbers underlying the data in hard-copy reports by using interactive software capabilities is critical to an understanding of the factors driving the patterns presented. The increasing popularity and accessibility of Internet technology holds promise not only for more efficient delivery but also of improved support for the dialogue that successful profiling initiates.

Support

Provider profiling is a process, not an event. The implications of this truism for data are seldom fully appreciated at the beginning of the effort. Support requirements fall into two categories. The first is a knowledgeable staff to respond to questions from those in receipt of a profile to answer questions, and particularly to pursue investigations of aggregate profile measures back through progressive levels of detail data to raw claim or encounter records. The second is staff to refresh the data sources and perform iterations of the statistical measures at agreed-on intervals. Again, if the principal objective is changing behavior, then one component of planning is to design the monitoring and evaluative mechanisms to establish whether changes have occurred.

Conclusion

It is imperative to identify and prioritize the profiling objectives to inform the selection of data, determine the analytic dimensions, and assess the scale and expense of resources for development, production, and support of the profiling effort. This must also include a sober assessment of the availability, scope, quality, and timeliness of data.

Conventional eligibility and enrollment data sources offer important information for planning profiles. Claim and encounter data can identify whether a medical event occurred and for what reason (diagnosis), and what services were delivered and why. Regardless of the profiling objective, the number and specificity of ICD–9 diagnosis and procedure codes, as well as the specificity of CPT codes, is vitally important to successful profiles. Medical groups embarking on their own profiling process should consider including ICD–9 diagnosis codes taken to a fourth or fifth digit to distinguish important acuity levels. All profiles should have some economic content. However, this is often a difficult issue for profilers because of the inconsistency of financial information. Increasingly, profiling analysts use RVUs in parallel with other financial data to help normalize their measures of resource value, whether or not they use RBRVS as part of their payment strategy. The scope of data required to support physician profiling and the way data are treated analytically vary substantially by provider, the provider's relationship to members and patients, and the analytic tools deemed appropriate for achieving the desired business objectives. The best PCP profiles consist of data on all the assigned members and data from claim and encounter systems from all providers for all types of care. Physician specialist profiles and comparative profiles of individuals and practice groups must be developed within the context of a peer group for each specialty and subspecialty. For analysis of profiling data, it is important to select the appropriate units of analysis. The quality of source data for the development of profiles is certainly a pivotal factor, but few data are intrinsically valuable. Rather, it is the entire process of planning, development and organization of the data, delivery of information, and follow-through that ensures management success.

Notes

1. Medicare uses the RBRVS to set payments, such as the Medicare fee schedule, for all services rendered to beneficiaries from Part B (nonfacility) providers, whether physicians, other professionals, or vendors. Each CPT code is assigned a total quantity of RVUs, which have three components: work, practice expense, and malpractice expense. Each component is adjusted independently and combined to a single RVU total value. Most analysts use either the full RVU unit to normalize resource units or only the work component. Although the system was developed with federal funds for use in the Medicare program, nearly all state Medicaid programs and much of the private insurance world uses it in modified form.
2. Adjusted Clinical Groups, formerly called Ambulatory Care Groups, were developed by researchers at Johns Hopkins University as a population-oriented measure of health status (illness burden) designed to be indicative of expected health care resource conception. These groups can be used to adjust for the differences in the illness burden of patient panels across providers or health plans. The software distributor is CSC Healthcare, Farmington Hills, Michigan.

   The Diagnosis Cost Group family of risk adjustment models was developed by researchers at Boston University and Health Economics Research originally to enable the Health Care Financing Administration to health-risk-adjust its payments to HMOs for Medicare beneficiaries. This methodology has been expanded to include models for the privately insured and Medicaid populations under age sixty-five. The distributor is DxCG, Waltham, Massachusetts.

CHAPTER THREE

HARVESTING DATA FOR PHYSICIAN PROFILING

The Administrative and Clinical How To's

Norbert Goldfield

In an ideal world, all clinically relevant information would be available for physician profiling. In fact, it is almost certain that within ten years, all relevant clinical information will be easily accessible to providers for physician profiling, at least for release internally. Obtaining clinically relevant information will not be the challenge. The challenge for providers, particularly physicians, will be to work together and to identify publicly acceptable methods of external release information. As Michael Millenson (1996) forcefully argues in his book in favor of public release, "How about driving out *my* fear each time I seek treatment from my profit-driven health maintenance organization (HMO), which has just signed up a joint venture consisting of a panic-stricken community hospital and a pampered group of local physicians who could not spell *capitation* a year ago if you spotted them all the vowels? That my friends, is fear."

Yet physicians also have a legitimate concern. Although public disclosure of comparative information is well established for managed care organizations and hospitals, there is little experience with public release of physician-specific information. As someone who has had experience with the approximately twenty states that produce hospital-specific mortality and severity profiles, I can attest to the difference between releasing information pertaining to a hospital with thousands of employees and releasing information pertaining to one physician or a small group of physicians. Simply put, the difference is one of public relations. Whereas large organizational entities such as hospitals, managed care organizations, and large medical groups either have or could have significant public relations resources to deal with the positive or negative fallout of the public disclosure of comparative information, small groups of physicians could not withstand such an onslaught. Yet physicians claim that currently available information is not scientifically valid and is not only inadequate in today's marketplace of ideas but denies patients information that would allow them to make better choices and to manage their own care better.

Although the challenges of external release are critical, harvesting available information represents a significant challenge. The key question physicians must face is how they can best obtain information regarding their practice that will have a measurable impact on the process and outcome of patient care. This chapter will examine this question, without being scientifically exhaustive, in the light of the current state of physician profiling and future research trends.

Desired Characteristics of Physician Profiles

Typically when a medical group decides to harvest data, the physicians in the group are focused on the task at hand, such as allocating income. But it is important to consider the manifold uses to which harvested data can be put. Thus, prior to harvesting data, a medical group should step back and consider the variety of uses of a physician profile. As part of this process, the medical group should consider the desired characteristics of physician profiles, whether used for internal or external purposes:

- Be of interest to as many consumers of physician profiles as possible (patients, employers, managed care organizations, and, of course, physicians themselves)
- Help to improve the process and outcome of care
- Have a firm basis in scientific literature while recognizing that much of clinical medicine is still an art and contains many controversies
- Meet certain statistical thresholds of validity and reliability
- Cost the minimum amount possible to produce
- Respect patient confidentiality and, if obtaining information from the medical record or using patient-derived information, obtain patient consent
- Ideally contain information on all patients the provider has in his or her case load, even patients who are technically on the physician's panel but have not been seen by the physician

The importance of addressing the needs of the various consumers implies an attempt to achieve political and scientific consensus between often differing and competing interests. This process to achieve consensus is just as important as the final product itself. In fact, successfully integrating the needs of differing consumers will result in a physician profile that has significant salience and importance that will improve both the process and the outcome of care.

Medical groups that want to harvest and then analyze their own data will have difficulty analyzing their entire patient case load unless they have access to a file, typically held by a managed care organization, that lists all the members of the case load—even those who may not have come to the physician's office at all in the previous year. Knowing about these patients is important from both a quality-of-care standpoint (for example, making sure that all patients have had appropriate preventive care tests) and also cost of services (such as setting the correct capitation rate).

It is important that physician profiles address both the outcomes and the processes of care. Several colleagues and I collected over one thousand patient responses to a questionnaire on desired characteristics of physician report cards (Goldfield and others, 1998b). Our analysis found that these patients (enrolled in three managed care organizations dispersed throughout the United States) valued information pertaining to the processes of care more than they valued information pertaining to the outcomes of care. In addition, while our knowledge pertaining to outcomes is continuously improving, patients appear to have very high confidence in and desire to have information pertaining to processes of care (such as availability of appointment times and friendliness of the staff).

Although the need for scientific validity for any data elements within a physician profile is obvious, the execution of such an effort is easier said than done. There are two dimensions to this important issue. First, from a harvesting point of view, only claims data on those patients who have come into the office are readily available to a medical group. The limitations of claims data are well known (and will be addressed in this chapter). Second, medicine is still very much an art and not a science. Physician profiling, particularly in the form of publicly available report cards, may give an aura of scientific validity, but medical groups and providers in general must emphasize the quality improvement and "art" aspects of both medicine and resultant profiles.

Consider the optimal treatment of diabetics, where differing points of view lead to a different emphasis on different aspects of diabetes care. These different emphases lead to the need to collect different types of data for provider profiles. Thus, some patients tolerate a lifestyle that includes frequent examination of blood glucose level and occasional hypoglycemic episodes; others prefer a lifestyle that might incur future complications in lieu of continuous glucose examination. Research has demonstrated that the role of patient interaction with the physician in this process is critical (Kaplan and Ware, 1995).

Results of patient satisfaction and health status measurement are increasingly available for providers. It is even technologically possible, though not commonly done, to integrate patient satisfaction data with information derived from a claims form. This combined information would allow the medical group to adjust patient satisfaction by severity of illness. As one might expect, from a clinical perspective, it is likely that sicker patients are less satisfied. A further step forward would be the integration of more sophisticated measures of severity of illness (such as the name of the pharmaceutical or the value of the outpatient result) together with claims or satisfaction data. However, laboratory results have not yet been integrated with claims and patient satisfaction.

Unfortunately, the "art" aspect of the science of medicine manifests itself when different clinical perspectives emerge even among different groups of medical professionals, as in the case of otitis media. These differences provide challenges to the need to achieve consensus on the data elements required for valid provider profiles. The challenge is even greater when considering the many consumers, especially physicians from different medical societies, who need to agree with the content and implementation process of physician profiles.

In the light of the increasing popularity of point-of-service plans, which allow the enrollee greater freedom of provider choice, the need for a sufficient sample size is a real and growing concern. The only practical means of dealing with this issue is for medical professionals to work together, alone or under the umbrella auspices of an organization such as the state medical society or national professional associations, and collect data until adequate statistical criteria are met.

There is at least one significant difference in the characteristics desired of physician profiles when used for internal purposes (private and confidentially to the physician) versus those used for external purposes: the threshold of statistical and clinical validity. The threshold does not need to be as high when physician profiles are used for internal quality improvement activities. The threshold for public release depends on the development of a communitywide approach to the need to release the information, a process for its release, and an understanding on how it will be used to improve both care and the doctor-patient relationship.

Data Elements Used in the Harvesting Process

A medical group desiring to profile member physicians always needs to ask the same question that must be applied to every administrative task: What will the information be used for? For the most part, physicians, like any health care institution, are most concerned about finances and increasingly interested in issues pertaining to quality. The following data elements are necessary for any harvesting efforts of data for any physician profiling objective pertaining to cost or quality:

- Unique patient identifier (often scrambled for patient confidentiality).
- Diagnostic information, typically provided using ICD–9–CM.

- Procedural information, derived from volume III of ICD–9–CM, CPT, and/or HCPCS codes. In addition, identifying information relative to the name of the pharmaceutical used is often present.
- Level of service information, such as that provided by evaluation and management CPT codes.
- Charges from services ordered by the physician and health care facility.
- Results of information derived from additional studies, such as patient satisfaction and measurement of patient health status.

Data Editing Process

It is likely that medical groups harvesting data will have an outside group process their data or have in-house expertise that will make certain that the data being processed are clean. It is important that physicians become aware of important data edits. The old maxim of garbage in and garbage out definitely applies to the data editing process. The data included in a physician profile are only as good as the effort the physician and other members of the health care team have made in completing the required data entry.

Among the most basic considerations in the data harvesting process are being sure that valid diagnostic or procedural codes (if present) are attached to each claim, valid charge information is included, and a valid patient identifier is present. Physicians and other members of the health care team may be interested in expanding the physician profile to encompass episodes of illness, a much more complex undertaking from every perspective. Two issues in particular merit emphasis: (1) a valid patient identifier that will allow linkage of various outpatient and possibly inpatient encounters and (2) a master member index (MMI) that reliably identifies each patient receiving care from a particular physician. Such an MMI would be able to ferret out whether John Smith is the same individual as John D. Smith.

The MMI issue is a significant one for medical groups because they often do not have access to a complete listing of all their covered patients. Typically the managed care organization or health insurer maintains this list. If the MMI is not available, the medical group is likely to profile on the basis of encounters for which they have data. Thus, without an MMI, the medical group will likely wish to profile, if possible, merged hospital and outpatient encounters; at a minimum, the medical group will wish to profile physicians and the medical group on just the outpatient encounters alone. However, relying on outpatient encounters alone should not be viewed as a long-term solution. For example, assessing the impact of a disease management program for congestive heart failure implies access to at least inpatient and outpatient encounters.

The issue of adequate sample size is significant. The ideal sample size depends on what the information will be used for. If the information is to be released to the public, the standard has to pass a much higher bar as compared to the internal release of information. Merging across diseases (such as hospitalizations) is almost always necessary because it is almost never the case that a physician has sufficient patients with any one diagnosis. It is important, after adjusting for severity of illness, to combine diseases at appropriate levels of severity. Thus, a patient hospitalized with a myocardial infarction (MI) with a high risk of mortality cannot simply be added with uncomplicated pneumonia patients. It is important for the medical group to inquire whether and how commercial vendors of severity adjustment and risk of mortality adjustment account for this issue and what algorithms they provide for merging data. A similar issue occurs on software packages that purport to profile across an episode of illness.

The data editing process for the profiling of episodes of illness is in fact much more complex. I recently participated in a large research project that developed a classification system for the measurement of episodes of illness. One of the most complex parts of the undertaking was the data editing process. For example, diagnostic data are refined and subjected to some basic edits:

- Diagnoses from nonprofessional providers, such as free-standing laboratories, ambulance services, and durable medical equipment vendors, were not retained because presumably they would replicate diagnoses from the physicians and institutions ordering the services.
- Physician diagnoses associated with inpatient services were discarded. These diagnoses should duplicate institutional data for the same admission, and the data from institutional sources are more reliable than data from physician offices.
- All diagnoses associated with an inpatient admission were retained. Only outpatient chronic diagnoses reported on two separate occasions were kept. Thus, except for a narrow list of diagnoses, the vast majority of diagnoses (such as chronic obstructive pulmonary disease) were required to occur twice before they were counted.

There are several efforts underway to look at episodes of illness, and different commercial offerings are available. Episode groups are classification systems categorizing illnesses through appropriately defined episodes of time. In broad terms, one must again ask what the objectives are of the medical group in desiring to profile episodes of illness. For example, episode treatment groups (ETGs) would be useful as a first cut of a large number of diseases, such as diabetes. Episode Grouper examines many of these same diseases but also profiles individuals with a combination of diseases (such as diabetes and congestive heart failure).

Harvesting Data

One has to crawl before one can walk. Similarly, a provider interested in profiling can harvest data in the following ways, presented in order of increasing difficulty from a technological point of view:

- Visit-based claims data from the inpatient sector
- Visit-based data from the outpatient arena
- Visit-based nonclaims data (such as patient satisfaction) from either the outpatient or inpatient sectors
- Linked outpatient data not linked to a master member index (or linked to a master member index)
- Linked inpatient and outpatient data not linked to a master member index (or linked to a master member index)

A provider who harvests any data at all typically examines data from one of the first three options. A number of forward-looking organizations are harvesting data from the last two options. Although these last two options are clinically and financially more desirable, most organizations are typically not able to harvest them for a variety of reasons, discussed below.

Medical groups will wish to harvest diagnostic information by episode of illness. It is important that they carefully evaluate the available software products that purport to measure clinically valid episodes. Individuals may have more than a single recorded diagnosis, for example. In this case, members of the medical group will want to know how the episode-of-illness software deals with patients who have multiple coexisting chronic illnesses. Many of these diagnoses will have no effect on future health care costs, others will indicate differing levels of severity of some underlying condition, and still others will indicate the presence of additional diseases. The technology should be able to distinguish at the individual level the importance of each diagnosis relative to an individual's health status. It should be sensitive to the whole constellation of an individual's diagnoses as well as the time frame in which they occurred. For example, angina occurring prior to a coronary bypass is unimportant because the bypass presumably will have resolved the angina for at least the immediate future. But angina that occurs after a bypass is very important because it means the problem either has not been resolved or has recurred.

Adjusting for Severity of Illness

When confronted with the need to examine quality of care and utilization of services, most physicians immediately parrot the age-old adage, "My patients are sicker." This conundrum needs to be addressed, and that can be done only by asking what the objective of the analysis is.

Case mix adjustments for purposes of quality improvement or utilization management represent only the first step in the quality improvement process. Physician profiles adjusted for case mix taken at one pinpoint in time should never be used to make final decisions regarding the quality or cost appropriateness of a physician's medical practice.

One of the most difficult questions facing a purchaser of a case mix technology is the degree to which the purchaser is comfortable with the use of potentially preventable complications as part of the severity adjustment logic. For example, with respect to myocardial infarction, many secondary diagnoses present on admission after an MI likely represent a comorbidity or sequelae of the MI. Thus if a patient develops complete atrioventricular block on the second day of admission, it is likely that this secondary diagnosis represents a comorbidity and not a complication. One could extend this analysis to a large number of other secondary diagnoses—with specific respect to MI.

A purchaser needs to answer the following question as part of the case mix purchasing process: Does the purchaser prefer a case mix technology that includes the potentially preventable complication in the logic? Such case mix logic gives the benefit of the doubt to the provider (hospital or physician). Without this decision, providers may be unfairly rated. Although my bias is to include all secondary diagnoses after admission, save for those that represent clear complications (the 9000 series of codes in ICD–9–CM), others might altogether reject such an approach. California is a leader in providing a middle ground: the collection of data of whether the secondary diagnosis was present on admission (*California Rules for Present Admission,* 1996). Such knowledge would allow the calculation of separate indices for all codes versus those codes only present on admission.

Types of Data Used in Current Physician Profiling

Claims-Based Data

There is significant experience with the use of inpatient claims data for physician profiling (Coulam and Gaumer, 1996). And although claims data are much maligned, they do have several advantages for quality improvement and utilization management purposes:

- With the implementation of diagnosis-related groups (DRGs), there is an extended period of experience with inpatient coding. More than twenty states have had the confidence to release to the public data on risk-adjusted mortality, length of stay, and charges using a version of DRGs, the APR-DRGs (all patient refined), which are adjusted for these dependent variables (Jones, 1996).

- Because of the significant financial issues at stake for the hospital, there typically is a considerable effort to code as accurately as possible.

- For enrollees with a chronic illness, who have the highest likelihood of interaction with the health care system, information pertaining to the quality of hospital care is likely to be very important.

- For at least one important aspect of quality within a hospital, mortality, the information is reliably coded and is of great importance to all consumers interested in physician profiles.

- For many physicians, there are sufficient numbers of patients for whom issues pertaining to quality and/or utilization can be examined. When that is not possible, there are statistical methods to aggregate clinically dissimilar patients into categories that have been adjusted for complexity.

- There is considerable experience with using claims-based data for quality improvement purposes, although this is still controversial (Weiner, Starfield, and Mumford, 1991).

A significant controversy still exists with respect to the validity of using claims-based data for quality improvement purposes. It is unlikely that the institutions and individuals who dismiss the validity of claims-based data for these purposes will change their minds. The best approach is two pronged. First, institutions and individuals who use claims-based data to improve quality need to continue to publish. More important, large organizations such as state health agencies and national centers providing input into data collection instruments such as ICD–9–CM need to include new data elements to increase the validity of claims data. For example, California mandates the collection of a data element indicating whether the secondary diagnosis on a hospital claims form was present on admission.

Over the past five years, researchers have begun to analyze claims data in sectors of the health care system other than the hospital. However, once again it is always important to clarify the objective for using claims data. There are two types of ambulatory care claims-based data: visit based and episodes of illness. With respect to visit-based ambulatory care–based claims data, profiling can provide information pertaining to utilization of services (provided that procedures are not a significant part of the case mix adjustment that is used to account for differences in severity of the patient's illness) (Shapiro, Lasker, Bindman, and Lee, 1993). So long as the objective is clearly specified, profiling can also provide information pertaining to quality of care provided to enrollees. Thus, the following types of information obtained from visit-based ambulatory claims data are useful for physician profiles for quality monitoring purposes:

- The presence or absence of a particular procedure (such as a vaccination or mammogram), the performance of which typically indicates that quality care has been provided for that particular condition
- The utilization of inappropriate site of care such as the emergency room for an asthmatic, which, if repeated continuously, may indicate an opportunity for improvement

According to a recent review of claims data used for physician report cards, "Despite their imperfections, claims data can be extremely useful probes to improve utilization, target continuing medical education, help manage complex patients, identify underserved patients and detect misprescribing as well as fraud and abuse" (Goldfield and others, 1998a).

We are at a relatively primitive state of physician profiling using claims data for episodes of illness. Significant enhancements will shortly appear on the market, including the development of severity-adjusted disease-specific categories with the following characteristics:

- Could be tracked over an episode of illness (Mitchell and others, 1996).
- Begin at hospitalization (such as a myocardial infarction) and track mortality over a ninety-day period.
- Identify procedure codes, which may represent a complication of care. The Center for Health Economics Research has identified the performance of a computed tomography scan shortly after discharge for an endarterectomy as a possible indicator of a complication of care (Schroeder and Lamb, 1996).

Patient-Derived Questionnaires

Two types of information are typically drawn from enrollees: satisfaction and health status. Although there has been no published information on the use of patient satisfaction questionnaires to improve physician performance, considerable anecdotal evidence points to the conclusion that such information is useful. I was involved in the development and use of a patient satisfaction questionnaire in a large staff model HMO. The results of this questionnaire were used as part of the salary increase for the staff model physicians. Of greatest importance, the physicians themselves were involved in the development of the questionnaire. From a cost point of view, it should be emphasized that patient satisfaction questionnaires do not require large numbers of enrollees to produce statistically valid information.

The last few years have seen the development of a significant number of well-validated questionnaires that measure patients' health status. The Foundation for Accountability, a competitor with the National Committee for Quality Assurance (NCQA) and Joint Commission for the Accreditation of Health Care Organizations, emphasizes improving outcomes, specifically health status (Lansky, 1996;

Brooks, 1995; Iezzoni, 1995). There appears to be little effort currently to add physician-specific profiles to its portfolio of profiling managed care organizations.

Encounter Data

Encounter-based data include any information drawn from the medical record and any other pieces of paper and or data files completed by a provider at the time of an encounter with a patient. With respect to inpatient profiling systems that use information drawn from the medical record, MedisGroups is the most well known (Brooks, 1995). Both hospital- and physician-specific profiles have been released to the public based on this risk adjustment system. The most extensive scorecard emanating from Pennsylvania is its "Focus on Heart Attack" (Pennsylvania's Declaration of Health Care Information). New York State has released physician-specific report cards in its analysis of hospital cardiovascular surgery since 1992 (Chassin, Hannan, and DeBuono, 1996). There is ample evidence to indicate that cardiovascular surgery mortality rates did decline as a consequence of the release of this information. However, the academic literature is controversial if the decline is only correlated with the release of physician-specific information or if other factors explain the decrease. According to a recent review of the New York State experience with public disclosure of risk-adjusted physician profiles, the developers of the report card declared, "We believe that the public release of data on mortality rates has played an important part in galvanizing physicians and hospitals to seize these opportunities to improve" (Chassin, Hannan, and DeBuono, 1996). However, there is no question that many experts have argued against this scorecard type of work. For example, individuals committed to quality improvement do argue that public release of this information instills fear into the providers of care, thus inhibiting commitment to improve.

Several medical specialty societies (urology, cardiovascular surgery) have also ventured into the field of physician profiles for specific hospital-based surgical procedures. Unfortunately many of these efforts are proprietary, and the developers have not opened the logic for scrutiny by independent researchers. Although it is difficult to evaluate the reliability and validity of these medical specialty society efforts, it is likely that such efforts will increase in importance. If the members of a specialty society are supportive of such efforts, it is likely that over time and after considerable internal development and release, these physician profiles will be publicly released.

Making the Choices

One of the main drawbacks in all of these efforts is the cost of obtaining this information. In addition, it would appear that there has been little involvement on the part of organized medicine. Rather, the business community is largely driving this process. Possibly it views this strategy of obtaining NCQA-based information as an intermediate step prior to direct contracting. The net result of such efforts will be the public release of physician profiles for at least a medical group of substantial size.

Faced with a bewildering array of choices, the medical group must decide which type of data to begin to use. The choice depends on the purpose. For purposes of internal release of data pertaining to cost and quality, claims data have significant acceptance in the medical market. Software packages are available that use claims data to profile medical groups on a visit encounter basis, ambulatory visits tied together into an episode, or, ideally, ambulatory visits tied together with hospitalization claims into a more complete episode. Occasionally purchasers demand that the medical group take patient satisfaction data into account. The advantage is that there are many commercial vendors for patient satisfaction products and that the associated cost is relatively low. Abstracting from the medical record should be done only if one has a very specific purpose in mind or is in the unfortunate position of having to work under the mandate of a purchaser requirement. Encounter-type data will become increasingly available as management information systems grow more sophisticated.

Future Data Availability for Physician Profiling

The future of physician profiling can be analyzed from two perspectives: the push for external release and the integration of disparate types of information, leading to a significant reduction in costs and simultaneous increase in validity for increasingly sophisticated physician profiles. With respect to the latter, increasingly sophisticated yet inexpensive physician profiles will be available in the short term. We are on the threshold of a revolution in lifting the electronic and organizational barriers to inexpensively linking salient elements for physician profiling. With respect to hospital-based care, many hospital-based systems will be able to link clinical and administrative data in the not-too-distant future, thus significantly increasing the power of the profiles for hospital-based services. Health care organizations are expending significant resources in an effort to link hospital and ambulatory care data. In the short term, advances in this area will result in a number of advances:

- A link between the name of the pharmaceutical and severity-adjusted claims data. This will increase the clinical validity of, for example, examining outcomes of care for diabetics. These databases are available now.
- A link with outpatient laboratory values. This will provide further clinical validity for the analysis, for example, of outcomes for diabetics.

- A link between patient health status and claims-based, laboratory, and pharmaceutical information.

The challenge will be implementation. Implementation is extremely difficult, and policymakers will need to pay attention to the following types of issues:

- Acceptance by individual physicians and all other consumers of the report card. Acceptance includes not only participation in the development of the profile but also an in-built quality improvement process to use the profiles effectively. We still understand very little about how consumers can best use these profiles (Edgman-Levitan and Cleary, 1996; McGee and Knutson, 1994).
- Protection of patient confidentiality.
- The development and implementation of new statistical and profiling techniques to enhance the validity of the physician profiles.

In the meantime, we need to have a strategy in place for current efforts to promote valid and reliable physician profiling.

A Forward-Looking Strategy

A strategy on physician profiling must deal constructively with issues of patient confidentiality and a research agenda on physician profiling.

Issues of Patient Confidentiality

Patient confidentiality can be ensured if strict policies are rigorously adhered to. In addition, encryption methodologies under development will facilitate patient and physician confidence in the confidentiality of physician-specific profiles (Goldman, 1998).

A Research Agenda

A research agenda on physician profiling is needed that does not paralyze physicians and policymakers into inaction. A forward-looking research agenda on harvesting of physician profiling data as it pertains to internal versus external release of physician-specific information would include at least the following questions:

- What topics are physicians and other customers interested in with respect to physician profiles? We should not assume that all patients are interested only in outcomes such as mortality. The harvesting of outcomes information other than mortality and certain complications almost inevitably must rely on information drawn from encounter data, a much more expensive proposition.

- What are the optimal methods to engage physicians and other customers in the development process of these profiles? Engagement of physicians can result in the harvesting of more accurate physician profiles.
- What new approaches, from both an informatics and a clinical perspective, can be developed to produce reliable and valid physician-specific profiles inexpensively? These new approaches need to include the determination of which organizational arrangements can facilitate the development and implementation of physician-specific profiles with adequate sample size.

Conclusion

It is appropriate to conclude this survey of the broad field of harvesting physician-specific reports by recalling the fate of one of the earliest efforts to produce these reports. Ernest Codman, a surgeon at the Massachusetts General Hospital, proposed that de facto physician report cards be developed and publicly released (Codman, 1990). This information was drawn from encounter data, all laboriously collected by hand. For these efforts, the Massachusetts General Hospital dismissed him from the staff, and the American College of Surgeons at their annual meeting burned his report cards in the fireplace of the hall where they were meeting at the Waldorf Astoria Hotel in New York City.

Seventy-five years later we still have a long road to traverse in our understanding of what type of physician-specific report cards we need; there remains considerable controversy. In the short term, medical groups will do well to use one of the commercial packages and harvest claims or patient satisfaction data. With respect to claims data, most medical groups will be able to use only claims data generated from a single visit. In the near term, this information will be useful for cost comparisons across and within the practice together with aspects of quality. A medical group that is more interested in quality will eventually need to harvest data that merge individual encounters into episodes of illness. A number of commercially available software packages are available that will allow the group to profile episodes of illness for quality of care, utilization, or capitation risk adjustment purposes. Early in the next century, medical groups will be in the blissful situation of being able to harvest, at low cost, data summarizing clinically detailed analyses of episodes of illness.

References

Brooks, D. C. "The Joint Commission on the Accreditation of Health Care Organizations." In N. Goldfield and D. Nash (eds.), *Providing Quality Care* (pp. 145–163). Ann Arbor, Mich.: Health Administration Press, 1995.

California Rules for Present Admission. Assembly Bill 3939, Chapter 1063. Statutes of State of California 1994, effective January 1, 1996.

Chassin, M. R., Hannan, E. L., and DeBuono, B. A. "Benefits and Hazards of Reporting Medical Outcomes Publicly." *New England Journal of Medicine*, 1996, *334*(6), 394–398.

Codman, E. A. "The Product of a Hospital, 1914." *Archives of Pathology Lab Medicine*, 1990, *114*(11), 1106–1111.

Coronary Artery Bypass Graft Surgery. *Pennsylvania's Declaration of Health Care Information.* Harrisburg: Pennsylvania Health Cost Containment Council, 1991.

Coulam, R. F., and Gaumer, G. L. "Medicare's Prospective Payment System: A Critical Appraisal." *Health Care Financing Review, Annual Supplement*, 1996, 45–76.

Edgman-Levitan, S., and Cleary, P. D. "What Information Do Consumers Want and Need?" *Health Affairs*, 1996, *5*, 42–56.

Goldfield, N., and others. "The Prospective Risk Adjustment System." *Journal of Ambulatory Care Management*, 1998a, *21*(2).

Goldfield, N., and others. "The Content of Report Cards: What Health Plan Members, Primary Care Physicians, and Managed Care Medical Directors Think Is Important." Unpublished manuscript, 1998b.

Goldman, J. "Protecting Privacy to Health Care." *Health Affairs.* Nov.–Dec. 1998, pp. 47–57.

Iezzoni, L. "Severity of Illness Measures and Assessing the Quality of Hospital Care." In N. Goldfield and D. Nash (eds.), *Providing Quality Care* (pp. 25–58). Ann Arbor, Mich.: Health Administration Press, 1995.

Jones, P. "Logic and Applications of the All Patient-Refined DRGs: The Greater Southeast Community Hospital Experience." In N. Goldfield and P. Boland (eds.), *Physician Profiling and Risk Adjustment* (pp. 299–316). Gaithersburg, Md.: Aspen, 1996.

Kaplan, S., and Ware, J. "The Patient's Role in Health Care and Quality Assessment in Providing Quality Care." In N. Goldfield and D. Nash (eds.), *Providing Quality Care* (pp. 59–82). Ann Arbor, Mich.: Health Administration Press, 1995.

Lansky, D. "Overview: Performance Measures—The Next Generation: Joint Commission." *Journal for Quality Improvement*, 1996, *22*(7), 439–442.

McGee, J., and Knutson, D. "Health Care Report Cards: What About Consumers' Perspectives?" *Journal of Ambulatory Care Management*, 1994, *17*, 1–14.

Millenson, M. L. "Public Disclosure: A Commentary." In N. Goldfield and P. Boland (eds.), *Physician Profiling and Risk Adjustment.* Gaithersburg, Md.: Aspen, 1996.

Mitchell, J. B., and others. "Using Physician Claims to Identify Postoperative Complications of Carotid Endarterectomy." *Health Services Research*, 1996, *31*(2), 141–152.

Schroeder, J., and Lamb, S. "Data Initiatives: HEDIS and the New England Business Coalition." *American Journal of Medical Quality*, 1996, *11*(1), S58–S62.

Shapiro, D. W., Lasker, R. D., Bindman, A. B., and Lee, P. R. "Containing Costs While Improving Quality of Care: The Role of Profiling and Practice Guidelines." *Annual Review of Public Health*, 1993, *14*, 219–241.

Weiner, J., Starfield, B., and Mumford, L. (1991). "Development and Application of a Population Oriented Measure of Ambulatory Case Mix." *Medical Care*, 1991, *29*, 452–472.

CHAPTER FOUR

SEEING THE FOREST THROUGH THE TREES

Developing Evidence-Based Profiling Reports

Suzanne Austin Boren, E. Andrew Balas, Kui Chun Su

The current debate over health care quality and the intensive search for more efficient methods repeatedly highlight the need for adequate technology assessment of clinical information services. New drugs cannot be marketed without demonstrating their efficacy and safety in controlled clinical trials. Yet clinical information service developers and physician executives are often forced to make decisions affecting health services based on speculation regarding benefits of various service changes instead of high-quality scientific evidence. The application of feedback techniques in managing health services illustrates the need for better evaluation and more data.

An American Medical Association survey indicated that more than one-half of physicians are subjects of clinical or economic profiling (Emmons and Wozniak, 1994). Profiling reports give providers direct comparisons of their performance with that of their colleagues. In spite of the frequently suggested potential and widespread use of information feedback, the results of before-and-after studies on profiling vary (Williams and Eisenberg, 1986; Parrino, 1989; Eisenberg and others, 1977). Some randomized clinical trials of such feedback indicate that physicians change their practice patterns after receiving the comparisons (Marton, Tul, and Sox, 1985; Reid, Hodges, and Drucker, 1977). Other trials have reported inconclusive or nonsignificant results (Wones, 1987; Steele, Bess, Franse, and Graber, 1989).

Information systems have become active ingredients of health services, but the assessment of the new information technology is still considered a controversial issue. Practitioners interested in applying the new information technologies need information on the results of clinical evaluation of computer systems. The shortage of reliable data on the practical value of information services probably contributes to the current underinvestment in health information technologies. Health care organizations invest, on average, only 2.6 percent of their operating budget in information technology, a marked contrast with the average 8 to 9 percent in banking (Smith, 1993).

Delineating and Locating High-Quality Evidence

In health sciences, not all types of published evidence carry the same weight. The HIV/AIDS guidelines of the Agency for Health Care Policy and Research (AHCPR) apply a three-grade system (randomized clinical trial or well-designed population-based study, other types of studies, and expert opinion) (El-Sadr and others, 1994). The Round Table Conference on Clinical Trials for the Treatment of Sepsis used three grades of recommendations with five levels of evidence (randomized trials with low false-positive negative errors, randomized trials with high false-positive and high false-negative errors, nonrandomized concurrent cohort studies, nonrandomized historical cohort studies, and case series) (Sibbald and Vincent, 1995).

The strength of recommendations and quality of evidence can be evaluated by applying the criteria set forth by the U.S. Preventive Services Task Force (U.S. Preventive Services Task Force, 1996; Woolf, DiGiuseppi, Atkins, and Kamerow, 1996). Studies supporting the intervention can be placed into one of the following categories according to study design: randomized, controlled trials; controlled trials without randomization; cohort or case-control analytic studies; multiple time series, uncontrolled experiments with dramatic results; and respected opinions, descriptive epidemiology.

Randomized clinical trials can be further scrutinized by assigning a trial quality score using a validated quality scoring tool. For example, a tool tailored for the quality evaluation of health services research trials has been developed and validated based on information from a variety of sources (Balas and others, 1995). The specification of quality aspects considers the recommendation of various textbooks and monographs on the methods of clinical trials, earlier published quality evaluation forms, and requirements of research synthesis including meta-analyses of clinical trials. This tool consists of twenty questions assessing site, sample, and randomization; process of observation; presented data; and statistical analysis.

Insufficient demonstration of effect of information interventions has been repeatedly criticized by evaluators of clinical computer applications. In a review of reports on clinical computer systems, over 75 percent of 135 articles were anecdotal, and only half of the remainder met basic scientific criteria for the conduct of clinical trials (Haynes and Walker, 1987). A basic shift is required in how scientists view research concepts as opposed to research results; the former are generally not considered proper objects for review or dissemination. Similar issues have been raised in other areas of health sciences. For example, a systematic review indicated that in only 10 percent of the reports were the conclusions of the investigators supported by the evidence they presented.

Although early evaluation studies focused on the accuracy of information generated by computer systems, newer studies tend to focus on differences in the process or outcome of care due to the information system. Randomized controlled clinical studies can provide the most valid information about the efficacy of computerized information systems in patient care (Balas and others, 1996a). Randomized controlled trials (RCTs) have achieved widespread recognition as sources of top-quality scientific evidence of the difference made by particular clinical interventions (Horwitz, 1987; Friedman, Furberg, and DeMets, 1985). If the study design, data collection, and analysis are well planned, RCTs can reduce the risks of selection bias, nonstandard definitions, missing data, and multiple comparisons.

Feedback: Balance Statement of Clinical Practices

There is certain confusion in the literature over the terminology used to describe clinical feedback techniques. Various types of information are presented routinely to health care providers (for example, profiling reports, feedback analyses, reminder checklists, and computer-generated alerts). Physician reminders, messages arriving at the time of clinical decision making, are sometimes called immediate feedback. True feedback, however, represents a report on past activities to influence future clinical decisions. It is a much-needed bridge between reminders and education.

Feedback programs can be divided into two major categories based on their dominant approach in the interpretation of practice patterns.

Feedback Based on Stated Objectives

The first category is feedback based on stated objectives. In quality improvement programs, measurable objectives are critical to drive everyone in the right direction and serve as mileposts against which progress can be gauged (Tenner and DeToro, 1992). Feedback programs can provide convincing evidence to encourage certain types of clinical action. In a family medicine center, a successful feedback program was implemented to encourage prescribing generic drugs (Gehlbach and others, 1984). During a nine-month feedback period, members of the experimental group received monthly computer printouts on their prescribing behavior for the preceding month. Whenever one of twenty-eight feedback drugs was prescribed by brand name, a message informed the physician about the generic equivalent and the potential cost savings. This intervention resulted in significant cost saving.

Feedback Without Specifying Objectives

Some feedback programs avoid specifying measurable objectives (Keller, Soule, Wennberg, and Hanley, 1990; Slomski, 1990). The provided information is restricted to the presentation of data without suggesting any interpretation. Usually the provider of the feedback information has some objectives (such as reduction in utilization rates), but these are not disclosed. This approach assumes that intriguing data stimulate physicians to define quality improvement goals and change practice patterns appropriately.

Usually feedback programs without stated objectives present data on variation in utilization rates, costs, outcomes, or adverse effects. For example, a series of interventions at a 228-bed general hospital provided physicians with feedback at regular intervals concerning the amount of laboratory services employed in treating their patients. Case-mix-adjusted estimates of laboratory tests allowed each physician to compare his or her use of tests with that of peers in the same department at the same hospital. The intervention resulted in a reduction of 1.8 tests per patient (Berwick and Coltin, 1986). Another study evaluated retrospective peer comparison feedback in containing hospital antibiotic costs (Parrino, 1989). Each month attending physicians in the top fifty percentiles for expenditure were notified of their status in relation to their peers. Over a year, no significant reduction in expenditure was noted. However, feedback without measurable objectives has obvious limitations in supporting corporate quality improvement programs and certainly cannot disseminate guidelines.

There is a widespread interest in using peer comparison feedback to shift the average utilization of clinical procedures by the members of a provider group. Based on the results of the several randomized controlled clinical trials testing peer comparison feedback, a multilevel meta-analysis was conducted to assess the clinical effect of peer comparison feedback interventions (profiles) in changing practice patterns.

Systematic computerized and manual searches were combined to retrieve articles on randomized controlled clinical trials testing profiling reports. Eligible studies were randomized controlled clinical trials that tested peer comparison feedback intervention and measured utilization of clinical procedures. To use all available information, data were abstracted and analyzed on three levels: (1) direction of effects, (2) *p*-value from the statistical comparison, and (3) odds ratio. The advantages of testing the same hypothesis in three slightly different sets of studies with three different statistical methods are that all valuable information can be captured from all trials and substantially different approaches can examine the same hypothesis. An analysis restricted to the odds ratio alone can lose the information from many trials with valuable information in the direction of the effect.

In the meta-analysis of this study, the average frequency of clinical activities was considered for the experimental and control groups. The statistical tests evaluated the hypothesis that the average performance of a provider group subjected to peer comparison feedback differs from the average of a similar but not subjected control group. The first level of analysis used a vote counting method in combining votes on the direction of effect of each study (Bushman, 1994). The sign test was used to determine whether the ratio of positive trials significantly exceeds the ratio expected under random variation. The second level of analysis used a *z*-transformation method to synthesize the *p*-value from individual trials. The overall *z*-value was calculated by summing the individual *z*-values and dividing the total by the square root of the number of trials eligible for this level of analysis (Hedges, Cooper, and Bushman, 1992). The third level of analysis used the odds ratio method to compare utilization (Peto's modification of Mantel-Haenszel method; Yusuf and others, 1985). In estimating odds ratios, 95 percent confidence intervals were calculated for the individual studies and for the combined effect.

The first level of the meta-analysis (vote counting) included all twelve eligible trials. Ten of the trials were positive, and two were negative. The significance level for the twelve trials was $p < 0.05$. In the second level of the meta-analysis (*z*-transformation), the combined significance test for eight trials resulted in an overall *z*-value of 1.98 ($p < 0.05$). The third level combined five trials. The five trials were heterogeneous (test for heterogeneity $X2_4 = 70.023$, significant). The primary effect variable in two of the five trials had a nonsignificant odds ratio because 1.000 was included in the 95 percent confidence intervals (see Table 4.1). However, when the five trials were combined, the overall odds ratio calculated with the Mantel-Haenszel method became significantly greater than 1.000 (1.091, CI: 1.045–1.136).

The results of this meta-analysis document a statistically significant, but quite modest, effect of peer comparison feedback on the utilization of various clinical procedures. A small utilization difference made by profiling can be observed over several months of an intervention period. Considering the small effect on clinical practices, it is unfortunate that profiling of physicians has become common practice before reliable validation has been made in randomized controlled clinical trials.

TABLE 4.1. FEEDBACK TRIALS.

Trial and Year	Odds	Ratio (95 Percent Confidence Interval)
Frazier and others, 1991	7.76	(CI: 7.36–8.26)
McPhee and others, 1989	1.16	(CI: 1.06–1.26)
Winickoff and others, 1984	1.29	(CI: 1.13–1.45)
Winickoff and others, 1985	1.05	(CI:-0.87–1.23)
Wones and others, 1987	1.02	(CI:-0.96–1.08)
All available trials	1.09	(CI: 1.05–1.13)

This meta-analysis indicates that peer comparison feedback alone cannot be considered a substantive quality improvement or cost-control intervention. However, in commonly encountered situations, peer comparison feedback is able to make a difference in less than 5 percent of patient-physician contacts. Consequently the potential cost saving effect of peer comparison feedback is unlikely to exceed the cost of the intervention for most clinical procedures. Such effort to control spending seems to cost more money than it conserves.

Randomized Controlled Trial of Clinical Direct Reports

Controlled studies indicate the marginal effect of profiling; other versions of feedback can be much more promising. A clinical trial examined the effect of linking practice data to published evidence (Balas and others, 1998a). The hypothesis of this study was that clinical direct reports (practice data with pertinent evidence from the literature) would influence the number of patients allocated to the peritoneal dialysis modality versus hemodialysis for the management of end-stage renal disease.

The randomized controlled clinical trial was conducted at five dialysis centers. All physicians caring for patients at the study centers were asked to participate. Many centers use a team approach to make treatment decisions, so the number of physicians was limited to those who make the ultimate decision as to treatment modality. Of the participating physicians, half were assigned through centralized computerized randomization to the intervention group, who received the monthly database report, and half were assigned to the control group, who received no report. Five of the ten physician participants were assigned through centralized computerized randomization to the intervention group, who received twelve center-specific clinical direct reports encouraging the consideration of peritoneal dialysis, and five were assigned to the control group, who received usual information but no similar report.

Twelve monthly clinical direct reports were generated from existing data, such as the Missouri Kidney Program (MOKP) database and the United States Renal Data System (USRDS) annual reports. The clinical direct reports combine center-specific information or practice patterns with the latest published evidence on the efficacy and cost of various dialysis modalities. The reports contained information in the form of quotations and tables covering the following areas:

- A center-based comparison for each trial center in the study compared to other centers throughout Missouri
- Current survival rates for patients, nationally and in Missouri, by treatment modality
- Current age, gender, and race distributions for all patients, nationally and in Missouri, by treatment modality
- Opportunities for cost saving, as illustrated through current studies in the literature
- Quality-of-life comparisons for patients on hemodialysis versus peritoneal dialysis
- Complication and hospitalization rates for patients in Missouri by treatment modality
- Information gathered from the trial database pertaining to the physician's patient population.

Reports were mailed to the intervention group with an explanatory cover letter and a stamped, self-addressed postcard to be sent back on receipt of the report.

One hundred fifty-two patients were eligible for monitoring. Table 4.2 presents the allocated treatments and reasons for the allocated treatments. The number of patients allocated to the less expensive but equally effective treatment (peritoneal dialysis) was significantly higher in the intervention group than in the control group (15.3 percent versus 2.4 percent). Patient preference was the most common reason provided for the allocated treatment (88.2 percent). Ninety-three patients (95 percent confidence interval: 79.5 to 104.3) in the intervention group and 41 patients (95 percent confidence interval: 29.1 to 53.8) in the control group indicated patient preference as the reason for the allocated treatment. Other specific reasons for the allocated treatment included family preference, residual renal function, medical need, and catheter failure. A significantly greater number of control group patients indicated patient preference as the reason for their treatment allocation ($p = 0.004$). A significantly greater number of intervention group patients provided other specific reasons for their treatment allocation ($p = 0.036$).

Due to a need for transient use of hemodialysis by some patients, the percentage of patients receiving peritoneal dialysis increased through the end of

TABLE 4.2. TREATMENT ALLOCATION IN THE DIALYSIS STUDY.

	Intervention Group	Control Group
Treatment allocation (start)		
Peritoneal dialysis	17 (15.3 percent)	1 (2.4 percent)
Hemodialysis	94 (84.7 percent)	40 (97.6 percent)
Reason(s) for treatment allocation		
Patient preference	93 (83.8 percent)	41 (100.0 percent)
Other specific reason	11 (9.9 percent)	0 (0.0 percent)
Reason not provided	7 (6.3 percent)	0 (0.0 percent)

the three-month follow-up (18.0 percent versus 4.9 percent, $p = 0.041$). There were no significant differences between the intervention and control groups in meeting patient preferences, metabolic status, and complication rates.

The results of this study show that communicating clinical practice statistics with appropriate comparisons and pertinent recommendations from the literature can be effective in changing practices. The homogeneity of intervention and control groups resulted from the randomization and was confirmed by the baseline comparison. Consequently the only detected difference at the end of the study, a difference in the use of peritoneal dialysis, should be attributed to the clinical direct reports applied in the intervention group. In more general terms, it is interesting to observe the significant effect of this nonintrusive, nonjudgmental, and simple information intervention on clinical practice patterns. The documented effect is in sharp contrast with the aggressive approach of many utilization management techniques that have never been tested in controlled experiments or showed questionable value in controlling rising health care costs.

Automated Generation of Individualized Feedback

Based on an expert system shell, the Quality Feedback Expert System (QFES) was developed to support clinical performance improvement through rule-based analysis of medical practice patterns and individualized distribution of published scientific evidence (Balas and others, 1996b). Through the application of direct mail and performance improvement concepts, the specific aims of the expert system development were to support the implementation of a wide range of clinical practice guidelines and improve patient care by informing physicians about clinical practice patterns and pertinent published recommendations.

The clinical direct report is defined as a confidential summary of clinical practice data and pertinent statements from research reports. It was primarily designed for practitioners whose practice data indicate substantial deviations from the guidelines. Figure 4.1 is a schematic representation of the entire performance improvement system that transfers clinical practice data and pertinent evidence from the clinical literature to the individual providers. The QFES development was based on an expert system shell that provided a flexible tool kit for rule-based generation of direct reports tailored to the needs of individual practitioners.

The system consists of three data and knowledge bases that can be revised and updated as needed. The quality parameter knowledge base stores a series of measurable clinical practice recommendations with substantiating evidence for each recommendation. Each parameter is defined by a brief description of the recommended clinical procedure (critical action), the condition making a population of patients eligible for the particular procedure, and a numeric target for the utilization rate of the procedure among eligible patients. Evidence from pertinent

FIGURE 4.1. QUALITY FEEDBACK EXPERT SYSTEM FLOW DIAGRAM.

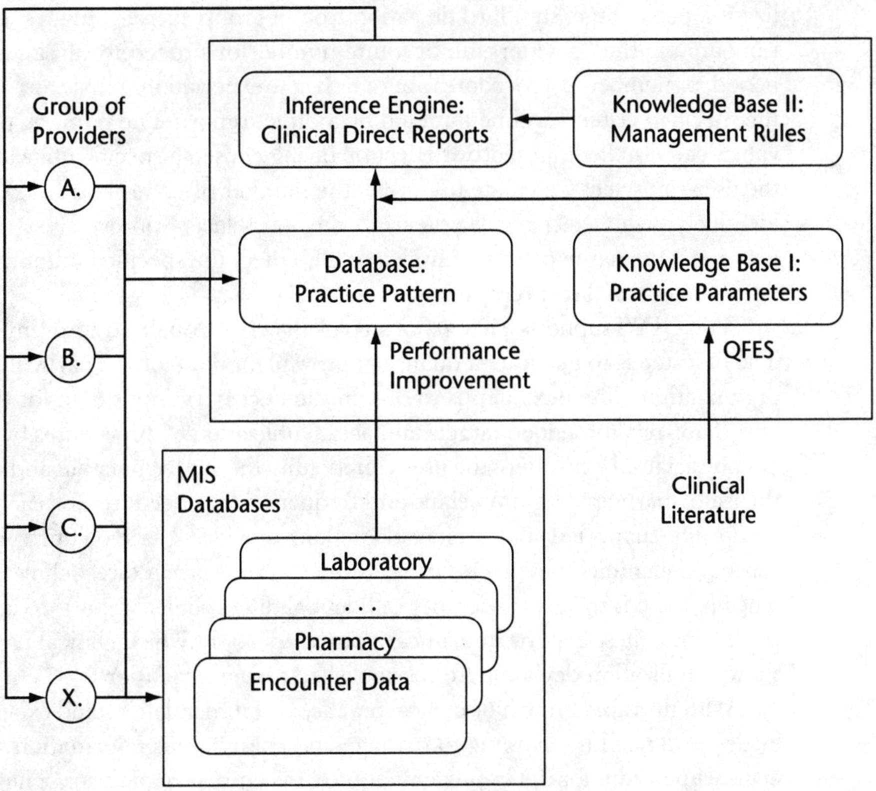

literature, accessed by clicking on one of the boxes for the five categories of evidence, is displayed in a smaller window. The parameters can be selected and copied into a quality improvement plan by the system user.

The practice pattern database stores data on the utilization of specific clinical procedures in various groups of patients. It provides information for the statistical analysis of patient care decisions by the participating physicians in the particular health care organization during the given period of time. The information enables the QFES system to compare expected and actual procedure utilization rates for each physician and identify variations in clinical practice patterns. The user can identify the source data file and examine or modify the list of participating physicians and frequency of procedures for each patient group. A key step of the collection of practice data is the Adjust function. Pressing the Adjust button ensures that the system keeps in the quality improvement plan only those parameters supported by actual practice data.

Finally, the management rule base consists of specific guidelines to identify physicians who should be targeted by a direct clinical report. The user can select an appropriate rule that can identify significant deviation based on a given utilization percentage, standard deviation from a group average, highest or lowest rank among the providers, an absolute number of procedures in an analyzed period, or number of procedures above or below expectation. Physicians who meet the specified criteria will be targeted by a direct report. The numeric threshold values can also be adjusted by the user. Having chosen a specific utilization rule, the user can select Calculate to display the number of physicians who would be identified by the selected rule criteria. If the user selects Approve, the system puts a mark by the name of those physicians who meet the specified criteria and will be targeted by a direct report.

The QFES supports each major step of the classic quality improvement cycle. The first step is to generate a quality improvement plan for the particular health organization. The next step is to obtain the necessary input data for the comparison of recommended targets and actual utilization of procedures by individual physicians. In this step, the user can identify the source data file and examine the list of participating physicians and frequency of procedures for each patient group. The supported analyses include ranking providers based on utilization measures and identification of providers who need to receive a direct clinical report. The final step is the generation of confidential direct clinical reports to individual physicians. These reports inform care providers about which clinical procedures showed utilization deviating from established recommendations.

With the rapid growth of clinical practice recommendations and experimental evidence, a need is emerging to manage and channel this information to physicians who need it for the improvement of clinical practice patterns. The application of expert system technology provides significant advantages and greater flexibility in the analyses of individual practice styles as well as influencing those practice styles through direct mailing. Unlike many other systems, the QFES does not require expensive program development for the implementation of new practice guidelines. New parameters can be easily entered by the user who can focus on the clinical issues of practice recommendations.

Selecting Evidence for Feedback Reports

It has long been assumed that the type of evidence contained in medical research literature has an influence on the manner in which physicians choose treatments, but the precise relationship is not well understood. Despite the constant efforts to influence them, physicians have rarely been asked their opinions regarding the presentation and usefulness of different types of evidence on practice patterns. A survey of 515 oncologists indicated that physicians' perceptions of the results of clinical trials tend to overestimate the therapeutic gain from the use of adjuvant chemotherapy for breast cancer (Rajagopal, Goodman, and Tannock, 1994). Currently most health care organizations use noninterpreted physician profiling and peer comparison feedback, which seem to have a negligible effect on actual clinical practices.

In the fields of marketing and political science, the means of using evidence and language to influence decision making has been the subject of many analyses. Although these fields are by no means equivalents of medicine, the successful manner in which they have analyzed the motivational impact of various types of evidence and language has some implications for managing the process of care. Certain descriptive words and phrases were found to create quantifiable distinctions in the minds of readers of marketing researchers, such that the phrase "a significant change" had a perceived value of 47 percent and "a substantial change" a perceived value of 34 percent (Scipione, 1995). Overall, negative information appears to carry more weight than equally extreme or equally likely positive information. Negative evidence is considered powerful not only in politics but also in many other areas of human information processing because people are more strongly motivated to avoid costs than to approach gains (cost orientation) and because negative information stands out against a generally positive background (Lau, 1982).

The goal of this study was to analyze the partiality of primary care physicians to six different classifications of clinical evidence, measure the perceived strength of various types of published evidence, and explore what exact type of evidence is likely to have the strongest influence on clinical practice patterns (Balas and others, 1998b). This study surveyed a sample of randomly selected primary care physicians in family practice, pediatrics, and internal medicine. Eligibility criteria included that participating physicians had been involved in direct patient care and the clinical area was primary care. Physicians were considered ineligible for the study if they were retired, in residency training, or not engaged in active patient care. The survey questionnaires were distributed to primary care physicians in the integrated health systems from Virginia Mason Medical Center in Seattle, Washington; Health Partners of Southern Arizona in Tucson, Arizona; and Good Samaritan Regional Medical Center in Phoenix, Arizona.

The survey used seven clinical areas and corresponding procedures as examples to investigate the effect of evidence type:

Diabetes	Retinal examination
Diabetes	Foot examination
Tobacco use	Counseling
Asthma	Patient education
Colon cancer	Screening for fecal occult blood
Congestive heart failure	Multidisciplinary intervention to prevent readmission of elderly patients
Arthritis	Gastrointestinal ulcer prevention for patients taking nonsteroid anti-inflammatory drugs

Each of the seven targeted clinical areas assumed an actual practice pattern and a need to improve utilization.

Seven versions of the questionnaire were developed, each containing seven clinical areas represented by a vignette. Each clinical vignette included hypothetical data on clinical practice patterns with peer comparison and one of the following seven types of evidence: (1) randomized controlled clinical trial, (2) uncontrolled clinical study, (3) cost-effectiveness study, (4) epidemiological study, (5) recommendation by a panel of experts, (6) locally developed recommendations, and (7) no evidence. To control the effect of clinical procedure on the preference regarding presented evidence, the sequence of evidence was rotated through seven versions of the questionnaire.

Attitudes about the presented types of evidence were measured on a six-point Likert scale:

1   Complete dissatisfaction with the presented evidence; the message provided was completely useless and the physician would not change practice style.

2   The message was somewhat useless.

3   The message was maybe useless.

4   The message was maybe useful.

5   The message was somewhat useful.

6   The evidence supplementing the report on practice data was extremely useful; the physician would definitely increase the use of the procedure in his or her practice.

Of the 147 family physicians, internists, and pediatricians who received the questionnaire, 76 (52 percent) responded to the survey. The physicians were twenty-nine to sixty-five years old and had been in practice for six months to thirty-five years. The overall average Likert score regardless of the evidence type was 4.65, with a relatively small standard deviation of ±.85. Table 4.3 shows the average Likert scores with standard deviation for the perceived strength of seven types of evidence. The subsequent Bonferroni pairwise comparisons showed that the evidence type of randomized controlled clinical trial was significantly superior to locally developed recommendations and no evidence. The results of the analysis of variance showed that the type of evidence had a significant influence, and so did the clinical area. There was also a strong interaction between types of evidence and clinical areas.

Beyond the anticipated outcome that randomized controlled clinical trial is the most preferred type of scientific evidence, the most striking result is that the widely used interpretation approaches, local recommendation, and no evidence received poor rating, and their perceived value is significantly lower than the value of controlled evidence. In other words, current management practices tend to rely on inferior and less convincing evidence in interpretation of clinical practice data. This survey also indicates that some sort of added evidence is the strong preference of most physicians. Preferences are also influenced by preventive care procedures and physician characteristics. The clinical specialty appears to influence

TABLE 4.3. LIKERT SCALE FOR PRESENTED EVIDENCE.

Type of Presented Evidence	Likert Score	Mean (± SD)
Randomized controlled trial	5.07	(± 1.14)
Clinical study	4.88	(± 1.28)
Cost-effectiveness study	4.77	(± 1.18)
Expert opinion	4.76	(± 1.10)
Epidemiologic study	4.51	(± 1.36)
Locally developed recommendation	4.39	(± 1.39)
No evidence	4.37	(± 1.53)

SD means standard deviation.

the perceived value of uncontrolled clinical studies. These observations have direct relevance to the implementation of practice guidelines and upgrading of decision support systems with evidence from the literature.

Conclusion

Not all feedback reports are created equal. Users have to apply evidence-based management to change clinical practices. Trying to do something intuitively appealing may be an attractive quick fix, but it is unlikely to yield lasting results. An approach based on the latest scientific results would probably consider the following guidelines:

- Uninterpreted data tables of practice patterns can make practice patterns more consistent but will probably not achieve the primary goal of feedback reports of improving average performance.
- The content and format of the feedback report should replicate one of those interventions that have been successfully tested in randomized controlled clinical trials. Exhibit 4.1 shows a feedback report.
- Since interpretation appears to be a critical part of any feedback report, careful selection of evidence is recommended. Preference should be given to those types of evidence that seem to be more persuasive for clinicians.

In an age when evidence-based clinical decision making is advocated and reimbursement for experimental treatment is routinely rejected, health care management cannot be an exception. The scientific standards of care can benefit patients when individual clinical decisions are made and when policies are formulated for a defined population. Fortunately, the scientific foundation for health care management is not just an aspiration. Quality evidence is already available for many organizational interventions, including various types of feedback.

References

Balas, E. A., and others. "The Columbia Registry of Controlled Clinical Computer Trials." In M. E. Frisse (ed.), *Proceedings of the Sixteenth Annual Symposium on Computer Applications in Medical Care.* New York: McGraw-Hill, 1993.

Balas, E. A., and others. "Methods of Randomized Controlled Clinical Trials in Health Services Research." *Medical Care,* 1995, *33*(7), 687–699.

Balas, E. A., and others. "Effect of Physician Profiling on Utilization: Meta-Analysis of Randomized Clinical Trials." *Journal of General Internal Medicine,* 1996a, *11,* 584–590.

Balas, E. A., and others. "An Expert System for Performance-Based Direct Delivery of Published Clinical Evidence." *Journal of the American Medical Informatics Association,* 1996b, *3,* 56–65.

Balas, E. A., and others. "Effects of Linking Practice Data to Published Evidence: A Randomized Controlled Trial of Clinical Direct Reports." *Medical Care,* 1998a, *36,* 79–87.

Balas, E. A., and others. "Upgrading Clinical Decision-Support with Published Evidence: What Can Make the Biggest Difference?" In B. Cesnik, A. T. McCray, and J. R. Scherrer (eds.), *MEDINFO.* Amsterdam: IOS Press, 1998b.

Berwick, D. M., and Coltin, K. L. "Feedback Reduces Test Use in a Health Maintenance Organization." *Journal of the American Medical Association,* 1986, *255,* 1450–1454.

Breslow, N. E., and Day, N. E. *Statistical Methods in Cancer Research: The Analysis of Case-Control Studies.* Lyon: International Agency for Research on Cancer, 1980.

Bushman, B. J. "Vote-counting procedures in Meta-Analysis." In H. Cooper and L. V. Hedges (eds.), *The Handbook of Research Synthesis.* New York: Russell Sage Foundation, 1994.

Byar, D. P. "Why Databases Should Not Replace Randomized Clinical Trials." *Biometrics,* 1980, *36,* 337–342.

Dickersin, K., Min, Y. I., and Meinert, C. L. "Factors Influencing Publication of Research Results: Follow-Up of Applications Submitted to Two Institutional Review Boards." *Journal of the American Medical Association,* 1992, *267*(3), 374–378.

Eisenberg, J. M., and others. "Computer-Based Audit to Detect and Correct Overutilization of Laboratory Tests." *Medical Care,* 1977, *15*(11), 915–921.

El-Sadr, W., and others. *Managing Early HIV Infection: Quick Reference Guide for Clinicians.* AHCPR Publication, no. 94–0573. Rockville, Md.: Agency for Health Care Policy and Research, Public Health Service, U.S. Department of Health and Human Services, 1994.

Emmons, D. W., and Wozniak, G. D. "Profiles and Feedback: Who Measures Physician Performance?" In M. L. Gonzalez (ed.), *Socioeconomic Characteristics of Medical Practice, 1994.* Chicago: American Medical Association, 1994.

Ewigman, B. G., and others. "Effect of Prenatal Ultrasound Screening on Perinatal Outcome." *New England Journal of Medicine,* 1993, *329*(12), 821–827.

Friedman, L. M., Furberg, C. D., and DeMets, D. L. *Fundamentals of Clinical Trials.* (2nd ed.) Littleton, Mass.: PSG Publishing, 1985.

Gehlbach, S. H., and others. "Improving Drug Prescribing in a Primary Care Practice." *Medical Care,* 1984, *22,* 193–201.

Haynes, R. B., and Walker, C. J. "Computer-Aided Quality Assurance: A Critical Appraisal." *Archives of Internal Medicine,* 1987, *147,* 1297–1301.

Hedges, L. V., Cooper, H., and Bushman, B. J. "Testing the Null Hypothesis in Meta-Analysis: A Comparison of Combined Probability and Confidence Interval Procedures." *Psychological Bulletin,* 1992, *111*(1), 188–194.

Horwitz, R. I. "The Experimental Paradigm and Observational Studies of Cause-Effect Relationships in Clinical Medicine." *Journal of Chronic Disease,* 1987, *40*(1), 91–99.

Howell, J. H., Flaim, T., and Lung, C. L. "Patient Education." *Pediatric Clinics of North America,* 1992, *39*(6), 1343–1361.

Keller, R. B., Soule, D N., Wennberg, J. E., and Hanley, D. F. "Dealing with Geographic Variations in the Use of Hospitals." *Journal of Bone and Joint Surgery,* 1990, *72A,* 1286–1293.

Lau, R. R. "Negativity in Political Perception." *Political Behavior,* 1982, *4*(4), 353–377.

Lomas, J., and others. "Opinion Leaders vs. Audit and Feedback to Implement Practice Guidelines." *Journal of the American Medical Association,* 1991, *265,* 2202–2207.

Magruder-Habib, K., Zung, W. W., and Feussner, J. R. "Improving Physicians' Recognition and Treatment of Depression in General Medical Care." *Medical Care*, 1990, *28*, 239–250.

Marton, K. I., Tul, V., and Sox, H. C. "Modifying Test-Ordering Behavior in the Outpatient Medical Clinic: A Controlled Trial of Two Educational Interventions." *Archives of Internal Medicine*, 1985, *145*, 816–821.

McNabb, W. L., Wilson-Pessano, S. R., Hughes, G. W., and Scamagas, P. "Self-Management Education of Children with Asthma: AIRWISE." *American Journal of Public Health*, 1985, *75*(10), 1219–1221.

National Asthma Education Program. *Executive Summary: Guidelines for the Diagnosis and Management of Asthma.* National Heart, Lung, and Blood Institute/National Institutes of Health. Expert panel report 1991; publication no. 91–3042A.

Parrino, T. A. "The Nonvalue of Retrospective Peer Comparison Feedback in Containing Hospital Antibiotic Costs." *American Journal of Medicine*, 1989, *86*, 442–448.

Rajagopal, S., Goodman, P. J., and Tannock, I. F. "Adjuvant Chemotherapy for Breast Cancer: Discordance Between Physicians' Perception of Benefit and the Results of Clinical Trials." *Journal of Clinical Oncology*, 1994, *12*(6), 1296–1304.

Reid, R. A., Hodges, A. G., and Drucker, R. P. "Utilization of Computerized Medical Data System to Assess and Improve Patient Appointment Keeping." In A. O. Wist (ed.), *Proceedings of the First Annual Symposium on Computer Applications in Medical Care.* New York: Institute of Electrical and Electronic Engineers, 1977.

Sacks, H. S., and others. "Meta-analysis of Randomized Controlled Trials." *New England Journal of Medicine*, 1987, *316*, 450–455.

Scipione, P. A. "The Value of Words: Numerical Perceptions Associated with Descriptive Words and Phrases in Market Research Reports." *Journal of Advertising Research*, 1995, *35*, 36–43.

Sibbald, W. J., and Vincent, J. L. "Round Table Conference on Clinical Trials for the Treatment of Sepsis." *Critical Care Medicine*, 1995, *23*(2), 394–399.

Slomski, A. J. "Cut Costs and Improve Care Too?" *Medical Economics*, Mar. 1990, pp. 48–53.

Smith, L. "The Coming Health Care Shakeout." *Fortune*, May 17, 1993, pp. 70–75.

Steele, M. A., Bess, D. T., Franse, V. L., and Graber, S. E. "Cost Effectiveness of Two Interventions for Reducing Outpatient Prescribing Costs." *DICP Annals of Pharmacotherapy*, 1989, *23*, 497–500.

Tenner, A. R., and DeToro, I. J. *Total Quality Management: Three Steps to Continuous Improvement.* Reading, Mass.: Addison-Wesley, 1992.

U.S. Preventive Services Task Force. *Guide to Clinical Preventive Services.* (2nd ed.) Washington, D.C.: U.S. Government Printing Office, 1996.

Weingarten, S. R., and others. "Practice Guidelines and Reminders to Reduce Duration of Hospital Stay for Patients with Chest Pain: An Interventional Trial." *Annals of Internal Medicine*, 1994, *120*, 257–263.

Williams, S. V., and Eisenberg, J. M. "A Controlled Trial to Decrease the Unnecessary Use of Diagnostic Tests." *Journal of General Internal Medicine*, 1986, *1*, 8–13.

Wones, R. G. "Failure of Low-Cost Audits with Feedback to Reduce Laboratory Test Utilization." *Medical Care*, 1987, *25*, 78–82.

Woolf, S. H., DiGiuseppi, C. G., Atkins, D., and Kamerow, D. B. "Developing Evidence-Based Clinical Practice Guidelines: Lessons Learned by the US Preventive Services Task Force." *Annual Review of Public Health*, 1996, *17*, 511–538.

Yusuf, S., and others. "Beta Blockade During and After Myocardial Infarction: An Overview of the Randomized Trials." *Progress in Cardiovascular Disease*, 1985, *27*, 335–371.

EXHIBIT 4.1. CONFIDENTIAL FEEDBACK
INFORMATION ON ASTHMA PATIENT EDUCATION.

Utilization Rates (in percentage)

Target rate	80–100
Group average (S.D.)	43 (+ or - 5)
Your practice pattern	35

EVIDENCE

Randomized controlled clinical trial

"Subjects in the experimental group completed a half-hour diagnostic interview, followed by four individually tailored 45-minute education sessions on the self-management of asthma. . . . In the 12-month post-education period, intervention group patients averaged 1.9 emergency treatments: the control group averaged 7.4 emergency treatments; treatments pre-education were 6.1 and 5.7, respectively. There was no difference in post-treatment non-emergency visits or drug scores between the two groups."

McNabb, W. L., Wilson-Pessano, S. R., Hughes, G. W., and Scamagas, P. "Self-Management Education of Children with Asthma: AIRWISE." *American Journal of Public Health*, 1985, *75*(10), 1219–1221.

Expert Recommendation

"Patient education involves helping patients understand asthma, helping patients learn and practice the skills necessary to manage asthma, and supporting patients for adopting appropriate asthma management behaviors and adhering to the treatment plan. Providing information contributes to but is not enough by itself to accomplish these objectives. Developing the patient's asthma management skills as well as the patient's confidence that the patient can control asthma is required."

National Asthma Education Program. *Executive Summary: Guidelines for the Diagnosis and Management of Asthma.* National Heart, Lung, and Blood Institute/National Institutes of Health. Expert panel report 1991; publication no. 91–3042A.

"Concomitant with increased understanding of the pathophysiology of asthma and the medications used to control the process has been a greater appreciation of the role of co-management or self-management. Several programs have been developed to help parents and children with asthma gain better control over the disease, thus decreasing morbidity and significantly improving quality of life. These programs are available to physicians and health care organizations, and it is strongly recommended that asthma education, both as a formal course and in the physician's office, be regularly incorporated into the care plan for every child with asthma."

Howell, J. H., Flaim, T., and Lung, C. L. "Patient Education." *Pediatric Clinics of North America*, 1992, *39*(6), 1343–1361.

CHAPTER FIVE

CASE MIX ADJUSTERS

Theory and Praxis

Manon Spitzer Ruben, Peter Braun, Philip Caper

A decade ago, physicians representing four New Hampshire and Vermont hospitals and communities met monthly for a year to investigate a twofold difference in local hospitalization rates for adult pneumonia. Each physician proceeded initially from the certainty that "my patients are sicker," whether the community's admission rate was relatively high or low. Patients do differ, of course, in both the number and types of medical conditions they experience and in the severity of each condition. Physicians differ too in terms of medical specialization, the selection of medical and surgical services they perform, and the medical characteristics of their patients. Case mix adjusters attempt to identify and account for such differences comprehensively, consistently, and systematically so that providers and provider groups can be compared fairly and paid equitably.

In 1986 in New England, the physicians had to identify and achieve consensus on qualifying diagnoses for pneumonia, criteria for severity and for relevant coexisting or complicating conditions, and indicators for hospitalization. Finally, they had to conduct a tedious chart review on each patient who had been hospitalized as well as on a random sample of patients treated in ambulatory settings but not admitted. Little of the required information was accessible in either standardized or electronic formats. Today case mix software systems rapidly address standardized, clinically oriented data from inpatient and all ambulatory settings. They systematically assess and measure differences in patients' health status, quantify the economic impact (financial risk) of "sicker patients," and normalize for differences in service mix (for example, between surgical and nonsurgical specialists).

Objectives of Case Mix Adjustment

In a managed care or fixed contract payment environment, the objective of case mix classification and adjustment is to enable physicians and other providers to provide medically appropriate care without financial penalty. The hope is that adjustment reduces incentives for risk aversion and underservice in managed care and for overservice in fee-based systems. Without such adjustment, some providers face unresolvable dilemmas between the ethics of their professions and fiscal solvency. This is well illustrated by the experience of an academic faculty practice group contracting with a state Medicaid agency to provide primary care medical management in their community. It soon became evident that the practice group was caring for two and a half times more HIV/AIDS patients—over three hundred lives—than any other contracted medical group. Without case mix adjusted payments reflecting the tenfold higher-than-average costs of this group, the practice faced bankruptcy.

Evolving Science of Adjustment

The first case mix systems sought to identify and explain variations in resource consumption retrospectively in order to provide a rationale for payments so that rates of increase could be both contained and made predictable. Payment-oriented case mix systems also had to facilitate adjustments for the introduction of new technology and changes in the costs of goods and services so as to reflect reasonably current experience and cultural values. Recently the concepts of case mix adjustment have been substantially extended to encompass the assessment of financial risk represented by a person's overall health status and to predict future expenses as legitimate reflections of medical needs. The science of risk assessment and adjustment is evolving rapidly and will undoubtedly accelerate as more clinically precise data describing health care experiences become available and generate new applications for payment systems and comparative analyses of provider performance.

Inpatient Systems

The first case mix adjusted payment system to achieve widespread success was the Diagnosis-Related Group (DRG), introduced in the early 1980s to implement a prospective payment system for inpatient hospital care under Part A of the Medicare program administered by the Health Care Financing Administration (HCFA). The DRG classification system was followed shortly by an "All Patient" DRG that provided additional classifications for age groups and medical conditions of more relevance to a nonelderly population.

Each DRG has a corresponding cost weight, which quantifies expected resource consumption. Complex procedures such as organ transplants and coronary artery bypass grafts have high cost weights because they place relatively high demand on time and staff of operating rooms, intensive care units, and other hospital resources compared to more common surgical procedures such as appendectomy and cholecystectomy, which have much lower cost weights. A typical patient with simple pneumonia or stroke does not require the same type or level of resource, so most nonsurgical admissions are also assigned relatively low cost weights. Tertiary care hospitals' average cost weight is generally higher than that of community hospitals because the latter's admissions consist of fewer complex surgeries and larger numbers of medical DRGs with relatively low cost weights. Cost weights are still the most commonly used value for case mix adjusting charges or payments and length of stay to create "apple-to-apple" comparisons for hospitals and hospital systems.

Controversy erupted immediately over the DRGs, with critics contending that the DRGs were insufficiently sensitive to patients' differing levels of severity and that the "sickest" patients within a given low-cost-weight DRG, such as congestive heart failure or stroke, also required exceptional resources, although of a different nature from that of complex surgeries. The private sector responded with new classification systems such as Disease Staging, Patient Management Groups, Medis-Groups, and the Acuity Index Method (AIM), among others. The public sector responded by enhancing the DRG classification system over time and developing Refined DRGs, All Patient Refined DRGs, and All Patient Severity Adjusted DRGs, which recognize differing levels of severity within a subset of DRGs. Although none of the commercial DRG alternatives achieved national recognition as the basis for a payment system and no consensus has ever developed on the merits of one or another of the methods (Iezzoni, 1997a, 1997b), they have been prominent in both hospital quality initiatives and health services research, especially between 1985 and 1995.

Ambulatory Systems

In the 1990s the Resource-Based Relative-Value Scale (RBRVS) enabled Medicare to set payments under the Medicare fee schedule for Part B (nonfacility) providers. Like DRGs for hospital care, RBRVS facilitates comparisons among providers based on standardized clinically relevant resource values. Commercial health plans increasingly use the RBRVS relative value unit (RVU) in provider performance profiles, independent of its use as a fee system. RVUs replace charged, allowed, or paid dollars where physicians operate in a mixed reimbursement environment and may be paid for the same services under different fee schedules. The RVU provides a constant value unit to reduce bias in comparative analysis of resource efficiency.

Comprehensive Systems

While payers continue to extend the applications of both DRGs and RBRVS out-side Medicare, a new generation of case mix adjustment systems is emerging. They respond to new information needs created by managed care rather than fee-for-service financing systems and to recognition that medical care for significant ill-nesses is multifaceted, involving sequences of events and providers. Unlike the DRG and RBRVS systems, which address only payments for component agents in a medical care delivery process, the newest case mix adjusters address broader population-based issues of medical and financial risk and changes in patients' health status over time. While these new systems share with the first generation of case mix classification systems a primary focus on creation of equitable payment strategies, they also offer valuable secondary applications with potential to improve the quality of care.

Next-Generation Adjustment Systems

Episode Treatment Groups (ETGs), an important and widely used software system for case mix classification and adjustment, combines features of the first billing-oriented systems like DRGs and the new patient-centered systems.[1] ETGs are an illness classification and episode-building methodology. Each episode measures patient resource consumption linking sites, types, and providers of service over time within a medical care model rather than a billing model. Clinically similar medical conditions are differentiated based on complications, comorbidities, and specific procedures. Although each ETG is clinically homogeneous, resource consumption between the start and finish of an episode often varies dramatically and is reflected in both cost differences and episode duration.

The ETG classification system alone is not designed to assess and quantify financial risk and predict resource use for populations. Research by the Codman Research Group (CRG) suggests that risk assessment tools can be integrated with episode analyses to explain much of the variation in expense and duration within the same ETG. The ETG classification system can also be used effectively to nor-malize case mix for provider comparisons, and ETGs are an important component of recent efforts to develop episode-based payments for selected procedures and for some physician specialties.

Risk Assessment and Adjustment Systems

The three case mix adjustment systems discussed in detail in this chapter—Ad-justed Clinical Groups (ACGs), formerly known as Ambulatory Care Groups,[2] Diagnostic Cost Groups (DCGs),[3] and the most specialized grouping system, the

Medicaid-focused Disability Payment System (DPS)—represent an important conceptual evolution (Kronick and Dreyfus, 1997). They all attempt to predict as well as to adjust for financial risk—that is, the economic consequences of differences in patients' health status and medical care requirement. All three are identified as population-based systems because they derive their predictive power from algorithms based on medical diagnoses and demographics recorded on each patient's claim and encounter data, supplemented in some cases by information on eligibility. Each system uses this information to predict resource consumption for populations or for individuals either concurrently or prospectively.

ACG, DCG, and DPS grouping methodologies and algorithms for prediction have been subjected to full disclosure, academic review, and publication. Their developers have the ability and commitment to the systems to maintain their currency and integrity regarding coding, changing technology and treatments, and new financial and organizational environments. All the adjustment and weighting methodologies are based on accepted statistical and epidemiological science and are regarded as both credible and unbiased (Dunn, 1995; Dunn and others, 1996).

Understanding the Environment for Case Mix Adjusters

Case mix adjusters, especially those that attempt to quantify and predict financial risk, do not operate in a vacuum. Adjustments to utilization and financial measures are always undertaken in relation to business objectives such as cost management or quality improvement. Case mix adjusters will be used most effectively when there is sensitivity to the environments in which they operate, the expectations and confusion they generate, and the data required for ensuring the integrity of the applications.

Setting Reasonable Expectations for Case Mix Adjusters

Substantial confusion still reigns in the managed care marketplace concerning case mix adjustment and the development of measures used for capitation rates, incentive payments, and quality and performance evaluations of health plans, provider groups, and individual practitioners. This confusion partly reflects the new information that needs to be addressed in managed care and most providers' relative inexperience with managed care. It also reflects the complexity of diagnosis-based systems, their need for accurate medical information based on administrative data, and lack of consensus on measures, terminology, and the objectives of case mix adjustment.

Any change in the way health care is financed changes the focus for accountability, the means by which it is measured, and the economic incentives for participation. The gradual shift to managed care has had a profound effect on the objectives of case mix adjustment. DRGs and RBRVS are designed to make payments predictable in a fee-for-service world. Accordingly the principal unit of resource value is a service event—in DRGs the hospital confinement, and in RBRVS each CPT code. In a managed care environment the unit of analysis is members or patients in aggregate populations for which a health plan or provider group assumes financial risk for all services or for substantial and defined components.

Some of the confusions arise in health plans and medical groups because case mix adjustment usually serves as both an insurance function and a quasi-medical function, and in each case imperfectly. The insurance function involves allocation of financial risk through some form of capitation arrangement or fixed payment contracting. The quasi-medical function is the application of case mix adjustment to comparative measures of physicians' utilization rates, costs, and intensity of treatment to evaluate the appropriateness of medical care patterns and cost-efficient practice styles.

Ideally the marketplace would like a system in which all risk is identifiable and predictable, all investment of resources affects financial risk quantifiably, and all influences on risk can be clearly identified, apportioned, and ascribed to an agent. Reality is nothing like that. The majority of health care events are acute and short term. For the minority that are predictable, the accuracy of those predictions is greater for population groups than for individuals. Joseph Newhouse and others have calculated that the maximum predictable component of a population's future medical expense is 15 to 25 percent (Newhouse, 1997). Much of this predictive power is based on a population's burden of chronic disease. One can more accurately predict future expenses for Medicaid-eligible Blind and Disabled, for example, than for Medicaid Temporary Assistance to Needy Families (TANF, formerly Aid to Families with Dependent Children). This is because the former by definition always consist of people with chronically disabling conditions of relatively known cost, and the latter include large numbers of young children whose experience of illness is essentially random.

Accepting and managing financial risk for a population requires a combination of insurance assumptions to cover the very large and unpredictable portion of health care expense and a case mix adjustment system that will identify, quantify, and predict the systematic component of illness-based expense. The best systems today are prospectively able to predict 8 to 12 percent of overall expenses, about half the theoretical maximum that Newhouse identified.

All the diagnosis-based case mix adjustment methods discussed here perform far better than age and gender adjustment alone. Typically, differences in the composition of a population's age and gender explain 3 to 5 percent of variation either retrospectively or prospectively (Dunn, 1995; Dunn and others, 1996). The actuarial assumption for a thirty- to thirty-five-year-old male is about $880 per year in medical expense. A thirty- to thirty-five-year-old male with HIV/AIDS has average expenses between $15,000 and $24,000 per year. The three systems discussed here perform eight to ten times better than age and gender for concurrent utilization and, depending on characteristics of the populations, three to four times better than age and gender prospectively.

Predictive accuracy declines with sample size for all methods. There are also differences in prevalence of medical conditions with known future costs between populations differentiated by geography, socioeconomic status, age group, gender, and other factors. Overall expense is more predictable prospectively for relatively small special needs populations with a high prevalence of strongly predictive conditions than for larger, younger, and more affluent populations with average health status.

Case mix assessment can be usefully applied descriptively to help characterize health status for any size group. Confidence levels for adjusting financial or other utilization expectations diminish substantially, however, for populations with fewer than two thousand individuals, regardless of the case mix grouping system.[4] These are limitations affecting every statistically based methodology, and they influence how far down—from plan to network to practice group to individual provider—one can reliably extend case mix adjustment to evaluations of performance or to risk-based financing.

What You See Depends on Where You Stand

Problems in communicating concepts of case mix adjustment often arise because managed care financing requires population-based statistical analysis. Most providers' perspectives, especially when the providers are physicians, are based on their interactions with members and patients, not populations. This difference produces tension over levels of applicability of case mix adjustment. All the case mix adjusters perform best relative to populations and least well predicting resources for an individual patient. Descriptively they offer valuable secondary benefits in identifying members with greater risk for high costs for enhanced care coordination efforts such as case management and disease management. Among the three systems discussed in this chapter, there are substantial differences in applicability based on group (population) size and on the objectives of case mix adjustment.

Morbidity Versus Severity

The case mix adjusters discussed here measure member morbidity: aggregate illness burden assessed from diagnoses drawn from multiple encounters across providers over at least six to twelve months. Morbidity is the appropriate measure for a health plan or medical group's insurance function. It is also valuable for some purposes from the perspective of good medical management, particularly for patients with chronic disease conditions. Many physician specialists, however, interact with patients only during periods of acute need. Their ideal for an adjustment tool is a measure that describes the acuity level of a specific medical condition during the term of the patient-physician interaction. With the exception of physicians in a primary care gatekeeper role, most physicians are also reluctant to accept predictions of utilization or cost that incorporate other providers' experiences (and expenses) with their patients. Providers ideally want a case mix adjustment system that documents the connection between the patients they know and how and why they are paid or evaluated with reference to other aspects of their performance.

Another set of problems arises related to the morbidity versus severity issue. Physicians usually view case mix adjusters based on administrative claim and encounter data systems as not sufficiently detailed and clinical. Physicians fault these sources as inadequate either because they are not designed to carry relevant medical information or because they are often inaccurately coded. In fact, because ACGs and DCGs aggregate information from multiple sources, ignore duplications of the same code, and concentrate on diagnoses that are the least discretionary and have the greatest predictive power, they avoid many pitfalls associated with procedure- and event-oriented approaches. No consensus exists on the requirements for development of a broadly applicable provider-oriented severity measure.

Data Preparation

Rigorous data evaluation is required before data are submitted for grouping by any case mix adjustment system. No methodology can totally overcome inadequacies of the basic source data. Systematic errors in data capture and quality are more difficult to detect and correct once grouping has occurred. This is because the groupers themselves use data elements selectively, aggregate, form decision trees, and apply weights to create hierarchies through behind-the-scenes processes that are inaccessible to end users.

In managed care settings, variation among provider groups in the completeness of data reporting, especially of evaluation and management encounters, is one of the greatest challenges to case mix adjustment. In extreme cases, some member populations may be represented to the grouper only by diagnoses associated with hospitalization, while others are also represented by a full spectrum of diagnoses common to ambulatory settings. When this occurs, an internally derived standard based on mean or median values is distorted, as are any comparative data, whether referencing internal or external standards. Little can be done in comparing such groups except to base comparisons on data restricted to what is available for all groups, which may be too limited for valid classification. Similarly, high plan turnover can play havoc with the best case mix adjusters. Members enrolled only briefly have had less opportunity to seek medical care and thus amass the claims on which case mix assessment and adjustment are based. Attempts to explain monthly as opposed to annual spending are also problematic because random or unpredictable events play a proportionately larger role in a shorter period (Newhouse, 1997).

The quality and quantity of ICD–9 coding is also important for differentiation between related medical conditions with specific complications that could influence resource requirements and morbidity scores. Analysts must choose financial data elements that are consistent with the financial arrangements of providers whose experience is to be case mix adjusted. Ironically the quality of clinical coding is relatively strong in fee-for-service because the transactional system bases payment on specific codes, and these are usually checked. In capitated systems incentives for complete documentation and accuracy are weak without the link to payment.

Standards and Peer Groups

Case mix adjustment implies selection of one or more standards for comparison and attention to the composition of peer groups. In general case mix adjusters work better for comparing larger groups than for individual physicians. One reason is that sample size is larger, which improves predictive power. Equally important, the medical "product" delivered to a patient of a specialty group—cardiologists, for example—is usually a composite consisting of a narrow band of services from two or three providers. In effect, the group is the provider, and as the focal point for analysis produces a more accurate representation of experience for case mix adjustment.

Understanding Adjusted Clinical Groups

ACGs were developed as a population-oriented measure of health status designed to be indicative of expected health care resource consumption. Originally intended for application only to the ambulatory setting and called ambulatory care groups, the grouping methodologies, embedded in state-of-the-art software, now address total resource consumption.

ACGs use claim and encounter experience for each member for a minimum of six months, and preferably one year. The grouper considers all ICD–9 diagnosis codes for all providers and settings except on laboratory and radiology claims, to avoid potential rule-out diagnoses, and on pharmacy claims. Users of the most recently released Version 4.03 have options to choose the method of classifying newborns, pregnancies, and deliveries based on the scope and quality of available data. Each individual's ICD–9 codes are mapped into ADGs (Adjusted Diagnostic Groups), which are collapsed to CADGs (Collapsed ADGs). The most frequently occurring combinations of CADGs become Major Ambulatory Categories (MACs), the first branches of the ACGs. MACs are subdivided into ACGs based on a patient's age, gender, and in many cases the total number of ADGs and the presence or absence of specific ADGs.

Every member or patient is assigned only one ACG, but may have any number of ADGs. There are no embedded normative values, although the developers have created and published a set of Resource Utilization Bands (RUBs) for each ACG. These are based on typical spending within that classification compared to the average member. Clients may use the RUBs either to set expected values or to compare to their own empirical results.

Most ACGs are not diagnostically homogeneous. Rather, diagnoses are grouped based on similarity of characteristics such as whether the condition is chronic, stable or unstable, likely to recur, and similarity of resource consumption. The Version 4.03 release introduces the concept of Major ADGs, eight ADGs found to be most indicative of high resource use. This increases the homogeneity of the ACG groupings with respect to resource expectation and, in many cases, clinical similarity as well. This enhancement is based on the empirical finding that among patients with multiple ADGs, some were of much higher cost than others. In addition, ACGs involving major diagnoses are split by age, distinguishing between pediatric and adult. Version 4.03 also greatly improves the grouper's classification of pregnant women and newborns, allowing analysts to assign the costs of delivery in a given year accurately and dissociate them from projections of future resource need. All told, these enhancements almost doubled the explanatory power for ACGs compared to Version 3.0 and virtually eliminated the difference between adjustment based on ADGs and ACGs.[5]

Susceptibility to bias in the ACG system is low. Frequency or volume of service, place of service, provider, and costs of specific services do not influence the assignment to an ACG or ADG, which is based exclusively on diagnosis. Because diagnoses from all providers are aggregated without regard to dates of service in the algorithms that form the ACG, and because most members who have substantial morbidity encounter many physicians, the coding patterns of a single physician are also unlikely to bias assignment substantially. In addition, none of the conventional incentives for upcoding applies because assignment is based on the aggregate experience, not a single event or service. Gaming the system requires both highly specialized knowledge of the grouper's logic and substantial collusion between providers.

As in any other statistical process, sample size always matters. The initial development of ACGs was directed toward nonelderly populations, and its objectives were not exclusively cost prediction; they included support for total resource planning and physician work load as well as medical management, such as predicting rates of office visits. Thus the architects of ACGs attempted to characterize the resource requirements of the full spectrum of needs represented by health plan populations. They identified but did not make their model's value dependent on only those with the highest costs. The ability of ACGs to characterize the anatomy and dynamics of health care interactions for typical health plan populations—providing metrics for routine care needs as well as interventions targeted on high-cost individuals—can be extremely helpful for delivery system management in addition to its application to capitation or financial incentive programs. Only a relatively few members are not classifiable to an ACG category, either because they did not access any health care providers or because the record of their encounter contained no codes indicative of any medical diagnosis.

In a study undertaken by the CRG covering two years of one state's Medicaid data representing nearly 800,000 individuals, only 8 percent failed to group to an ACG. By contrast, 40 percent did not classify into a Hierarchical Condition Category (HCC) in the Diagnostic Cost Group case mix system.[6] (See Figure 5.1.) This means that ACG classification for assessment and adjustment objectives can be used to help explain resource variation in relatively small populations. Many provider profiling applications involve populations of two hundred to five hundred members or patients, as do employer group analyses. Although ACGs were not designed to predict any particular service—that is, a single CPT procedure or a hospital admission for a specific medical condition—they can be applied to predict rates for classes of service such as total inpatient days and total ambulatory visits.

Research with ACGs reveals consistent adjustment results applied to at-risk populations such as PCP member panels, employer groups, and network segments for populations as small as 250, although 500 or greater is much preferred. There is also remarkable consistency between health maintenance organization (HMO) and provider preferred organization (PPO) health plans in the overall distribution of risk among their members, based on aggregations of members by ACG into levels representing progressively higher morbidity (see Figure 5.2). Results are similarly consistent in applications to physician profiles of primary care specialties

FIGURE 5.1. CLASSIFICATION OF MEDICAID WELL AND ILL.

Adjusted Clinical Groups

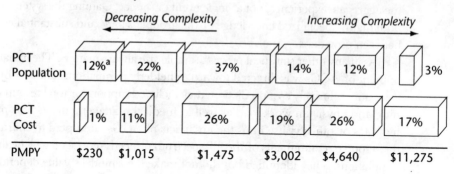

Diagnosis Clinical Groups

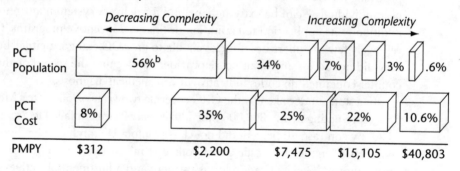

PMPY = Per member per year
PCT = Percent

Source: Codman Research Group.
[a]Eight percent are unclassified.
[b]Forty percent are unclassified.

and referral specialties that are evaluation and management oriented, that is, non-surgical.

One way of compensating for small sample size in provider profiling is to aggregate ACGs into morbidity levels. Each morbidity level is assigned adjustment weights based on commonalities in the average resource consumption of members in the ACG clusters. Each member is assigned to one ACG, and each ACG is assigned to only one morbidity level. Based on research on large and varied data

FIGURE 5.2. CLASSIFICATION OF
COMMERCIAL PPO AND HMO GROUPS, WELL AND ILL.

Adjusted Clinical Groups

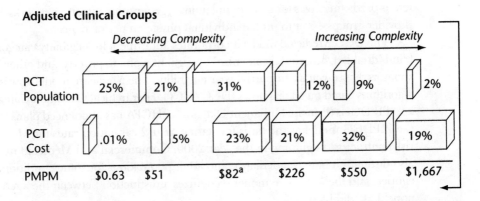

Source: Codman Research Group.

[a]Plan average, $93.

sets representing some 2 million lives, CRG has developed grouping recommendations and weights for morbidity levels for commercial, Medicaid, and Medicare populations. As in DCGs, the case mix adjustment application for these can be strengthened by incorporating eligibility status for Medicaid and Medicare, including disability. CRG has also developed illness burden values—a relative health status score—for individual ACGs based on the number of ADGs, the age and gender of the individual, and whether major ADGs are present.

Understanding Diagnostic Cost Groups

The DCG system is a family of health-based and profiling methodologies. The DCG model for Medicare was developed initially to enable the HCFA to risk-adjust its payments to HMOs for beneficiaries. Later, models were developed and tested for commercially insured nonelderly and for nonelderly Medicaid populations. All the models are contained in DCG Version 3.0, released in May 1998.[7]

DCGs use the demographics and diagnoses recorded on administrative claim and encounter data to predict the relative resource use of individuals either concurrently or prospectively. Unlike the ACGs, which attempt only to project total costs for populations, the DCGs also attempt to predict total costs at the individual patient level for both concurrent and future consumption. Such patient-level information can be used to identify the need for disease management programs in specific populations and patients who are candidates for case management interventions. The developers' principal objective for this case mix adjustment system is predicting costs for large populations—geographic regions, networks, large provider groups—not to profile individual physician performance.

The DCG Medicaid model incorporates adjustment for eligibility category—blind/disabled, other medically needy, pregnant women, poverty, and other state sponsored—as well as for partial year eligibility. The Medicare model consists of algorithms based on all diagnoses (DCG/HCC–Hierarchical Condition Category) and PIPDCGs (Principal Inpatient Diagnoses). HCFA has announced plans to use the PIPDCG model as the basis for setting Year 2 capitation rates for Medicare risk contractors beginning in the year 2000. Commercial and Medicaid models also distinguish between pediatric and adult populations for some condition categories, and the Medicare model recognizes a distinction between the aged and nonelderly disabled.

Every ICD–9 code from all clinicians' encounters is mapped by the grouper into 546 Diagnosis Groups (DGs) based on clinical homogeneity. These are then organized into 136 Hierarchical Condition Categories (HCCs), which consist of DGs that are clinically related and similar with respect to resource consumption. Each person may have multiple HCCs, but an individual's DG can map to only one HCC. These HCCs are the basic unit for case mix adjustment. These are further collapsed into 30 Aggregate Condition Categories (ACCs), which are used only for summarized reporting.

Not all HCCs are used for prediction, and concurrent and prospective models use different subsets of HCCs, distinguishing between diagnoses that are likely to have recurring resource use and those that are not. Some conditions that represent considerable cost in one year—for example, minor injuries; ear, nose, and throat disorders; and benign neoplasms—are not likely to produce costs in the next year. Other conditions—chronic diseases such as diabetes mellitus and major diseases like metastatic cancer—have a high probability for continuing high costs.

An individual patient may have multiple HCCs but receive only one risk score. The risk score indicates the absolute level of predicted total expenses for that individual, in a range from $200 to over $70,000 per year. An early DCG model uses the single highest-cost condition to predict subsequent year costs; Version 3.0 uses multiple condition models (HCCs) to capture the cumulative effect of multiple conditions on costs. These scores are summarized in preformatted reports by the software for user-defined subgroups, such as regions or counties, local networks, employers, and product lines. Whereas the preformatted reports are oriented toward the developers' interests in cost predictions, analysts can dissect the grouped data, provided in a detail-level output file, to identify members of interest based on the total high-cost projections, or by cost condition.

DCG grouping software embeds normative values for each DCG/HCC. However, users can also adjust the benchmark comparisons to apply actual local values and compare them to DCG-predicted levels. DxCG documentation specifies the source of normative values: Paid Dollars for Medicare, Paid Dollars for Medicaid, and Covered Charges for commercial insurance. Because DCGs correspond to fixed dollar amounts and the development data sets are now somewhat dated, especially for Medicaid, the dollar increments for the normative standard can be translated into current-year dollars by using an appropriate medical expenditure index as a weighting factor.

The explanatory power of DCGs applied concurrently to explain variation in total resource expense is similar to that for ACGs. For commercial populations, the most comprehensive model accounts for 39.56 percent of variation between groups, 43.18 percent for Medicare, and 35.91 percent for Medicaid populations. Prospective accuracy is more difficult to compare because no data have been published on ACGs for Version 4.0. DCGs' power to predict total expense prospectively is greatest for Medicaid in test populations. It predicted 23.1 percent of variation in total second-year costs based on current-year data, more than twice the percentage achieved for Medicare (8.5 percent) and commercial (9.4 percent). This should not be surprising, since for many segments of the Medicaid population, eligibility is based on a known medical condition and need, reducing its component of randomness relative to commercial and Medicare populations.

Like ACGs, DCG assignment is unaffected by volume of claims, the number of times the same diagnosis appears, site, or cost of service, so potential for bias is equally low. The DCG system's creation of HCCs also reduces the potential to reward a health plan or provider for coding more information. This is because costs associated with the highest-cost category condition subsume those for lesser conditions if more than one is represented. A small number of procedure-based categories are also created, principally for life-sustaining procedures such as tracheostomy. They are provided only for descriptive profiling and are not used in the adjustment algorithms.

DxCG researchers recommend DCG risk adjustment for setting and adjusting capitation rates, profiling provider resource use, and measuring provider efficiency controlling for case mix. The size of the provider group, health plan, or plan segment is extremely important, however. The power of the predictive algorithms, especially for prospective application, derives from serious medical conditions that occur relatively infrequently. The smallest population for which data are presented in DxCG documentation and research papers is 19,819 lives, of whom 4,960 had no claims or valid diagnoses in the sample. Prevalence is extremely low among the HCCs that have the strongest predictive power either concurrently or prospectively. In CRG's recent state Medicaid study, for example, prevalence for Metastatic Cancer (HCC005) is 19 per 10,000 compared to the DCG Medicaid benchmark of 23/10,000, and for High Cost Cancer (HCC006) the rates are 26 per 10,000 and 30 per 10,000 eligibles, respectively.

Because the DCG system is new to the commercial market, no good operational benchmarks are yet available to set minimum population thresholds for provider profiles. It appears unlikely that it will become a physician profiling tool as understood in today's marketplace, even for referral specialists. It is certain to have high value in predicting future resource use for budgeting and business planning to estimate future financial requirements for large populations, whether all enrolled members in a state or region, large network or provider group, or insurance product.

These caveats regarding population size are offset to a high degree by the value of the descriptive data produced by the DCG system at the individual member level. These data may be used to make decisions about allocating resources to provider units, identifying high-cost cases for management, and designing benefit packages for employer groups and others.

Understanding the Disability Payment System Model

Development of a Disability Payment System (DPS) classification model allows Medicaid to implement health-based payment where traditional methods used to set capitation would inadequately discourage plans from avoiding the type of high-cost individuals represented by people with disabilities. Architects and supporters of the DPS model, R. Kronick and T. Dreyfus (1997), argue that states will have to provide appropriate resources to providers and health plans to encourage innovation and quality. If they wish to pay appropriately without affecting the overall budget, they must use a payment system capable of differentiating between plans that enroll a disproportionate share of persons with above-average needs and those that do not. They must equally differentiate among low-, moderate-, and high-cost conditions among those that qualify an individual for disability status.

People with disabilities on Medicaid are an extremely diverse group. Many who receive Medicaid assistance because of disabilities such as mental retardation and mental illness do not require extensive medical care. Others have moderate, high, or very high costs as represented in the expenses associated with quadriplegia, AIDS, and hemophilia. According to data gathered by Kronick and Dreyfus on Medicaid recipients with disabilities in Ohio (see Figure 5.3), 49 per-

FIGURE 5.3. TOTAL DISABLED MEDICAID POPULATION.

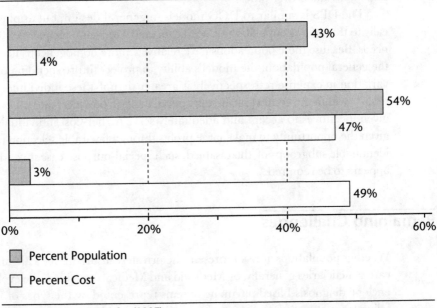

Source: Kronick and Dreyfus (1997).

cent of the disabled recipients accounted for just 3 percent of that group's total expenditures in 1992. At the opposite end of the spectrum, 4 percent of the disabled population represented 43 percent of total costs at an average exceeding $20,000 per recipient per year.

There is also a broad spectrum of costs represented by individuals within a disability category. For some, specificity of diagnosis coding is sufficient to distinguish cost levels. Among the skeletal and connective tissue diseases, for example, juvenile arthritis and osteomyelitis are high cost though relatively infrequent. Rheumatoid arthritis, disc disorders, and congenital leg deformities are seven times more frequent but average one-sixth the annual cost of juvenile arthritis and osteomyelitis.

Because these conditions are chronic, prediction of future costs by prior expenditure works extremely well; high-cost recipients in one year generally continue to have high costs in the next year. For purposes of case mix adjustment, DPS developers recommend classification of individuals into cost categories for estimating the following year's expenses. This approach has two virtues: it allows for payment for that individual on enrollment, so that plans that accept higher risks have immediate resources for meeting their needs, and it provides a cushion for the inevitable differences between individuals within a cost category and for the same individuals over time.

The DPS is similar to DCG models in general design, but applies specifically to that subset population of Medicaid (and Medicare) recipients with special needs. Because these populations have relatively more homogeneous need than in the general population, the model's ability to project future spending or explain variation in expense retrospectively is greater than if these individuals are considered within the context of the total population. If providers and plans are to be given incentives to accept and adequately serve higher-cost individuals but not given the opportunity to make large profits through favorable selection of readily identifiable subgroups of the disabled, such special-purpose case mix adjustment appears to be required.

Remaining Challenges

Whether populations at risk represent the privately insured, Medicaid and Medicare beneficiaries generally, or Medicaid and Medicare disabled, the evolving science of diagnosis-based payment systems represented by the types of case mix adjustment approaches described here directs provider groups and health plans away from seeking easy profits by avoiding risks and toward the achievable goals of improving value. The challenges posed by managed care incentives will not be surmounted by these systems alone. Rather, plans, providers, and researchers must simultaneously improve measurement sciences for assessing access and quality to ensure that improvements in budgetary management have no insidious and unintended consequences as price pressures inevitably rise.

Conclusion

The objective of case mix classification and adjustment is to enable clinicians to provide medically appropriate care without financial penalty. Appropriate case mix adjustment tools reduce incentives for risk aversion and underservice in managed care and for overservice in fee-based systems. Case mix adjusters will be used most effectively when there is sensitivity to the environments in which they operate, the expectations and confusion they generate, and the data required for ensuring the integrity of the applications. In managed care settings, variation among provider groups in the completeness of data reporting, especially of evaluation and management encounters, is one of the greatest challenges to case mix adjustment. Thus, rigorous data evaluation must be the first step, before data grouping.

In summary, ACGs are a population-oriented measure of health status designed to be indicative of expected health care resource consumption. The DCG system is a family of health-based and profiling methodologies developed to enable Medicare, Medicaid, and commercial managed care to project future payments based on members' current risk. The DPS classification model allows Medicaid to implement health-based payment where traditional methods used to set capitation would inadequately discourage plans from avoiding the type of high-cost individuals represented by people with disabilities.

Notes

1. Episode Treatment Groups are developed and marketed by Symmetry Health Data Systems, Phoenix, Arizona.
2. Adjusted Clinical Groups, formerly called Ambulatory Care Groups, were developed by researchers at Johns Hopkins University as a population-oriented measure of health status (illness burden) designed to be indicative of expected health care resource consumption. ACGs can be used to adjust for the differences in the illness burden of patient panels across providers or health plans. The distributor is CSC Healthcare, Farmington Hills, Michigan.
3. The Diagnostic Cost Group (DCG) family of risk adjustment models was developed by researchers at Boston University and Health Economics Research originally to enable the Health Care Financing Administration (HCFA) to health-risk-adjust its payments to HMOs for Medicare beneficiaries. The DCG methodology has been expanded to include models for the under age sixty-five privately insured and Medicaid populations. The distributor is DxCG, Waltham, Massachusetts.
4. See Appendix F of the *Guide to the Diagnostic Cost Groups (DCGs) and DxCG Software* (Release 3, SAS Version, Waltham, Mass.: DxCG, May 1998) for tables of confidence intervals relative to sample size associated with the DCG models applied to Medicare, Medicaid, and commercial populations.
5. Regressions for a number of health plans are shown on page B-14 of the "Guide to the Johns Hopkins University Ambulatory Care Croup (ACG) Case-Mix-Adjustment Software," March 1997, CSC Healthcare, Inc., Decision Technologies, 34505 West Twelve Mile Rd., Suite 300, Farmington Hills, MI 48331.
6. For further information concerning this ongoing research, contact the authors at the Codman Research Group, Andover, Massachusetts (e-mail: MRuben@Codman.com).
7. *Guide to the Diagnostic Cost Groups (DCGs) and DxCG Software*, Release 3 SAS Version, May 1998, available from DxCG, Inc., 411 Waverley Oaks Rd., Suite 330, Waltham, MA 02154.

References

Dunn, D. L. A Comparative Analysis of Methods of Health Risk Assessment: Final Report. Society of Actuaries, 1995.

Dunn, D. L., and others. "A Comparative Analysis of Methods of Health Risk Assessment." Paper presented to Codman Research Group, Andover, Mass., Apr. 1996.

Iezzoni, L. "The Risks of Risk Adjustment." *Journal of the American Medical Association*, 1997a, *278*(19), 1600–1607.

Iezzoni, L. (ed.). *Risk Adjustment for Measuring Health Care Outcomes*. (2nd ed.) Chicago: Health Administration Press, 1997b.

Kronick, R., and Dreyfus, T. *The Challenge of Risk Adjustment for People with Disabilities: Health-Based Payment for Medicaid Programs. A Guide for State Medicaid Programs, Providers, and Consumers*. Princeton, N.J.: Robert Wood Johnson Foundation, 1997.

Newhouse, J. "Risk Adjustment and Medicare: Taking a Closer Look." *Health Affairs*, 1997, *16*(5), 26–43.

Newhouse, J. *Risk Adjustment: Where Are We Now?* Washington, D.C.: Robert Wood Johnson Foundation, 1998.

PART TWO

HOW TO USE PROFILING DATA

CHAPTER SIX

USING PROFILING DATA

Facts or Fancies

Theresa A. Ryan-Mitlyng

Profiling is the process of measuring physician work and the outcomes it achieves. Depending on how close the measurer is to actual patient care activities, the view of physician work will vary. Although physicians frequently view profiling as intrusive, when it is done properly, it can serve as an opportunity for physicians to learn more about their work, allowing them to select areas to improve. To do that, physicians need information that accurately reflects their work—credible information that can be used to lead them to change their behavior in a way that positively affects patient care. Profiling offers an opportunity to physicians "by emphasizing the importance of improving outcomes through the process of information exchange and provider education" (Rosenstein, 1995). Physician profiling is becoming an area of great interest to many different parties:

Accrediting organizations

Employers and other purchasers

Hospitals

Independent practice associations (IPAs)

Medical groups

Payers, insurers, and managed care organizations

Patients

Physician hospital organizations (PHOs)

Physicians

Teaching and research institutions

The public and government

In order for physicians to survive and thrive in today's environment, they must become knowledgeable about their work. A noted physician stated, "I suggest that physicians try to get profiled and insist that the organizations in which they work or the systems of care in which they see patients invest in staff and information systems to profile them" (Ruffin, 1995). Physicians themselves should want to know what will help them succeed in practice so that their patients' health is improved and they are satisfied with their care. When this is the case, physicians are more likely to enjoy successful, productive, and rewarding careers.

The basic question is, What information on physician work really makes a difference? How helpful is all of this scrutiny? In profiling, what information will be so compelling that physicians will be willing to change how they care for patients? Out of all the information received from the insurance companies, from the hospitals, and perhaps from the practice group, what adequately reflects physician work? Will the information help determine better ways to treat patients and reduce costs? In evaluating profile data, what information is fact and what is fancy?

Solberg, Mosser, and McDonald (1997) write that "many clinicians have become uncomfortable with any effort to create measurement systems. That is unfortunate because measurements are absolutely essential to efforts for improving the processes of medical care." The question is why many clinicians are uncomfortable. In fact, most physicians are concerned about their performance and want to know how they compare to their colleagues. Careful profiling can give them good information on their performance and will allow them to make choices on how to improve.

Nevertheless, generating data capable of serving the intended purpose is no easy matter. Physicians who receive data based on incorrect assumptions about their work will disregard them. If the data do not clearly reflect the reality of physicians' work as they understand it, they will disregard the data. And they will disregard data presented in a form that is unusable or very difficult to interpret. Properly done, however, physician profiling offers the opportunity to establish correct and important information and to communicate it to the physicians and serve them as a resource. The key to useful profiling is to involve the physicians in the process from the beginning. It is the only truly acceptable way to ensure that the gathered data are based on evidence. Bell (1996) notes that in the selection of a profiling system, "Physician oversight allows for better understanding of the profiler's value in truly reflecting clinical practice." Four points are critical issues in performing physician profiling:

- Understanding how physicians deliver care before deciding what to measure
- Choosing the data that best reflect that element of physician work to be profiled, which requires an understanding of computer systems
- Presenting profiling data in a form that facilitates correct interpretation
- Understanding that measurement alone can affect physician behavior and thus the system of care in which they work

---

Understanding How Physicians Deliver Care Before Deciding to What to Measure

Part of the problem with physician profiling relates to gathering data based on incorrect assumptions. Not having a good understanding of how physicians work may lead down the wrong path and result in gathering data that are not helpful as shown in this sample.

A community hospital administrator has been asked to look at reducing the length of stay where possible. The administrator decides to examine variations in length of stay for patients with pneumonia who have been admitted by the primary care physicians on staff at the hospital. The data include a list of these physicians and the number of patients each has admitted. Also available are the diagnosis, admission date, and discharge date for each patient. The assumption is that the admitting physician is also the treating physician, and therefore the data will reflect each physician's work.

The results, set out in Table 6.1, show that the average length of stay for the entire staff is 2.9 days per patient. One physician, Dr. Kahn, had only one patient and this single patient stayed 7 days, giving Dr. Kahn an average length of stay (ALOS) of 7 days. Several other physicians had many more admissions each and a lower length of stay for their patients.

What the data do not show is that ten of the physicians are in a group practice and have a system of shared patient care. Five of the ten physicians have volunteered to be the "hospitalists" for their group, each rotating through the hospital for one week every fifth week, caring for all the group's hospitalized patients during that time. The rest of their time is spent in the office. Their call responsibility is every fifth night, and they handle all the admissions that come in for the group in the evenings and during the night. Because the hospital physicians cover the hospital call at night, they may get a disproportionate number of hospital admissions compared to the other physicians in the group who are based full time in the office. The hospital does rounds on all of the patients daily and writes all of the orders for the diagnostic workup, treatments, and consultations. In addition, the other five physicians in the group who work only in

TABLE 6.1. AVERAGE LENGTH OF STAY BY ADMITTING PHYSICIANS FOR PATIENTS WITH PNEUMONIA.

Admitting Physician	Patient	ALOS	Admitting Physician	Patient	ALOS
Dr. B. Allen	2	3 days	Dr. K. Palmer	6	3 days
Dr. S. Kahn	1	7 days	Dr. J. Jacob	8	2 days
Dr. H. Wallace	5	4 days	Dr. M. Wilson	2	4 days
Dr. P. Murray	7	3 days	Dr. W. Johnson	5	3 days
Dr. T. Baker	2	2 days	Dr. G. Fisher	6	2 days
Dr. D. Thompson	3	5 days	Dr. P. Adams	1	4 days
Dr. M. Ryan	5	2 days	Dr. M. Miller	2	2 days
Dr. L. Gipson	4	4 days	Dr. F. Bologna	7	2 days
Dr. J. Patrick	2	5 days	Dr. J. Strand	1	5 days
Dr. J. Lyons	8	2 days	Dr. P. Boland	4	4 days

TOTALS: 81 patients, 237 days, or 2.9 days on average for group practice physicians; 4.0 days on average for other physicians

the ambulatory setting may admit a patient from their office, but do not follow the patient on the hospital ward. These physicians have telephone contact with their partner in the hospital to follow the progress of the patient, but do not see the patient again until a follow-up visit in the office after discharge. Table 6.2 highlights the physicians in the group practice.

The average length of stay for the physicians in the group practice is 2.3 days as compared to an average of 4.0 days for the other physicians on staff. It appears that this group has developed a way of caring for patients that has resulted in a reduced hospital stay on average.

As new group practices form and solo practices become less common, the systems of care are changing too. Old assumptions about care also must change. How does a source outside the physician group factor in the realities of a group practice? Also, how does one include other factors that affect the measurement that has been chosen, such as comorbidities? Learning more about Dr. Kahn's practice reveals that she cares for patients with immune deficiency disease, and this particular patient was kept in the hospital for stabilization before being transferred to a hospice. To accomplish this type of transfer, multiple patient resources working in a coordinated fashion are needed, which can add time to the length of stay. In this example, the physicians might respond better to a hospital that looks at other factors over which the hospital itself has control, such as the length of time it takes to admit and discharge a patient, the length of time before antibiotics are started

TABLE 6.2. AVERAGE LENGTH OF STAY BY ADMITTING PHYSICIANS IN GROUP PRACTICE FOR PATIENTS WITH PNEUMONIA.

Admitting Physician	Patient	ALOS	Admitting Physician	Patient	ALOS
Dr. B. Allen	2	3 days	**Dr. K. Palmer**	6	3 days
Dr. S. Kahn	1	7 days	**Dr. J. Jacob**	8	2 days
Dr. H. Walla	5	4 days	Dr. M. Wilson	2	4 days
Dr. P. Murray	7	3 days	Dr. W. Johnso	5	3 days
Dr. T. Baker	2	2 days	**Dr. G. Fisher**	6	2 days
Dr. D. Thomp	3	5 days	Dr. P. Adams	1	4 days
Dr. M. Ryan	5	2 days	**Dr. M. Miller**	2	2 days
Dr. L. Gipso	4	4 days	**Dr. F. Bologna**	7	2 days
Dr. J. Patri	2	5 days	Dr. J. Strand	1	5 days
Dr. J. Lyons	8	2 days	Dr. P. Bolan	4	4 days

TOTALS: 81 patients, 237 days; 2.3 days on average for group practice physicians; 4.0 days on average for other physicians

Note: The ten physicians in the group practice are highlighted.

after admission, the length of time before a social services consultation is available for a patient requiring transport to another facility, and data on the comorbidities the patients present with that could explain longer length of stays.

In looking at a single element of physician work, physician profilers must understand the processes used to care for patients before deciding if this element is the appropriate one to measure. Too often a measurement is chosen first, and then much effort goes into figuring out what the results mean. Before beginning to measure and to avoid getting information that is not useful, profiling staff should check the accuracy of the assumption. They should test the assumption with those who have knowledge about the system that is being measured before starting the project. They also need to have in mind how physicians will use the data and determine if the data will be helpful and meaningful for that purpose.

Following is another example of gathering information before having a good understanding of the system in which the care is provided—this time in an ambulatory setting.

A physician practice has five members: two family practice specialists, two pediatricians, and one obstetrician. This small group practice is part of a larger group practice consisting of 150 physicians who work in twenty-five different offices. This particular practice works in an office located in a town ten miles from the main center. The practice schedules patients through a computerized scheduling system that is used across the entire group practice. The practice is staffed with one medical assistant per provider, a registered nurse who serves as the office manager, and shared front and back office personnel.

Patient access has become an issue of concern. The regional administrator has been receiving patient complaints that they cannot get appointments for routine exams or illness in a timely fashion with the family practice. The administrator decides to look at how many total hours of scheduled time are available and how many open slots are noted in a given period of time to see patients. These open slots will come from failed appointments or because there was an excess of physician availability in the schedule to see patients who requested care during that period.

The computer reports these slots as a percentage of time that is open in the physicians' scheduled hours. Without examining each individual doctor's schedule, it would be easy to assume that their schedules are the same. Encounter data for the practice as a whole are available, but the administrator did not choose to look at the data for the individual physicians in the report. He is trying to decide whether to hire another physician to increase access at this office. Table 6.3 shows his initial report.

What the administrator does not know is that Dr. Atkinson is very strict and will only schedule fifteen-, thirty-, and sixty-minute appointments. He does many routine physicals, spending an hour on each of those visits. He is not inclined to add same-day appointments and tends to have his schedule fully booked out six weeks in advance. His patients are happy about getting in for routine physicals and follow-up visits but are unhappy because he is rarely available to see them when they are sick; a few have written complaint letters to administration. His medical assistant will triage patients to his partner or to the urgent care clinic at the central office if he has no openings. Because of the restrictive nature of his practice, he tends to see the same number of patients each day and has very few open slots. In fact, on the rare occasion that he does add a same-day appointment, he often has to double-book it or put it into a slot where a patient canceled, thus appearing to be more than 100 percent filled. His profile generally shows a very small percentage of open time. On the surface, this may suggest

TABLE 6.3. PATIENT ACCESS REPORT FOR FAMILY PRACTICE PHYSICIANS.

	Scheduled Hours	Percentage Filled	New Patients	Transfers
January	304	95	40	10
February	270	97	45	15
March	236	96	37	23
April	300	92	33	35
May	270	98	40	28
June	270	91	38	16
July	218	97	29	19
August	200	92	25	23

that he cannot provide any more access for patients. He has chosen to limit taking new patients because his schedule is mostly full.

His partner, Dr. Brighton, likes to see acute care patients and has developed a schedule that has shorter time slots representing ten-, twenty-, and forty-minute appointments. He limits the number of longer, routine exams he will do in a day and leaves about 30 percent of his time slots open for same-day appointments. Dr. Brighton sees many more patients each day than Dr. Atkinson does, but because of the nature of his scheduling plan, he bears a higher risk to having open slots that do not fill. His patients complain that they cannot get in for a routine physical in a timely fashion, but they are very pleased that he is almost always available to see them when they are sick or injured. His profile consistently shows him at 90 to 100 percent filled. During illness season, he may occasionally see more than the designated slots, thus being more than 100 percent filled. The assumption may be that he has excess capacity much of the year and should be able to see more patients. He consistently sees about 25 percent more patients than his partner does. He takes new patients into his practice eagerly, but some have complained to the administration that they cannot get in for routine physicals very easily. Exhibit 6.1 illustrates a typical day of scheduled patients for Dr. Atkinson and Dr. Brighton.

EXHIBIT 6.1. TYPICAL DAILY SCHEDULE FOR DR. ATKINSON AND DR. BRIGHTON.

Dr. Atkinson			Dr. Brighton		
	Patient Name	Type of Visit		Patient Name	Type of Visit
8:00	Jones, Edna	New pt. H&P	9:00	Simon, Taylor	WCC 2 mo
8:15			9:10		
8:30			9:20	Fernandas, Mia	Annual gyn
8:45			9:30		
9:00	Sexton, Thomas	Pre-employ Px	9:40	Mellor, Mary	Diabetes
9:15			9:50		
9:30	Bretsky, Richard	Headaches	10:00	Webb, Joseph	Ear pain
9:45	Brooks, Sarah	BP check	10:10	Lai, Cecilia	URI
10:00	Phillip, Kirsten	WCC 5 yr	10:20	Esteve, Tony	Ear pain
10:15			10:30	Aitken, James	Suture rem
10:30	Fletcher, Joy	WCC 2 mo	10:40	Pentland, Alena	Cast check
10:45			10:50	Johnson, Robert	Sinusitis
11:00	Wilson, Errol	Arthritis	11:00	Tatla, Lena	Cough
11:15	Miller, Ethyl	Cough	11:10	Main, Clara	Knee injury
11:30	Schned, Tanya	Sinusitis	11:20	Ramos, John	Eye injury
11:45	Hanson, Joseph	F/U knee inj	11:30	Moore, Jill	Laceration
12:00			11:40		
			11:50	Rush, Jennifer	URI
			12:00		

EXHIBIT 6.1. TYPICAL DAILY SCHEDULE FOR DR. ATKINSON AND DR. BRIGHTON. *(continued)*

Time	Patient	Reason		Time	Patient	Reason
1:00 1:15	Peters, Kristine	Annual gyn		1:00 1:10	Janzen, Erica	Newborn
1:30 1:45	Mitchell, Susan	Diabetes		1:20 1:30	Lin, Joanna	WCC 2 mo
2:00 2:15	Kay, Johnathan	WCC 6 mo		1:40 1:50	Gilman, Phillis	Annual gyn
2:30 2:45	Marks, Glen	Physical		2:00 2:10	Ungar, Brian	Pre-employ Px
3:00	Doskotch, Walter	BP check		2:20		open
3:15	Pegler, Sandra	Back pain		2:30		open
3:30	Hersee, Phil	Thyroiditis		2:40	Olson, Jessica	Wrist injury
3:45	Herst, Cosima	Rash		2:50	Mitchell, Jeff	URI
4:00	Speers, Neil	Foot pain		3:00	Eschenbach, Kim	Eczema
4:15	Pilon, Marianne	Annual gyn		3:10	Arnold, Cynthia	Allergies
4:30				3:20	Rayter, Daryl	Headaches
4:45	Diamond, Rachel	Cough		3:30		open
				3:40		open
				3:50	Laughlin, May	Fever
				4:00	Sproule, Tiffan	Cough
				4:10	Hogan, Margaret	Ear pain
				4:20	Hoft, Grant	Ankle injury
				4:30 4:40	Morello, Stuart	Laceration
				4:50	Elliott, Marcia	Fever

Patients Seen	21		Patients Seen	29	
Scheduled Time	480 min.		Scheduled Time	420 min.	
Open Time	0		Open Time	40 min.	
% open time	0		% open time	9.50%	

The problem in this setting is that the patients' needs are met by how the physicians are scheduled. If both of the physicians in the group were like Dr. Atkinson and both appeared to have nearly 100 percent filled schedules, the administrator may decide there is a need to hire another physician to meet the patients' needs, especially if sick patients are not given access. If both of the physicians in the group were like Dr. Brighton and there was consistent open time in the schedule on a daily basis but a backlog of physicals, the administrator may determine a need to hire someone to take new patients and be available to do more physicals. Estimating the access in the care system based on one data element—percentage of open time—

is not enough. It is important to understand thoroughly the physicians' work that produced the data.

Redesigning the work load of the physicians and better matching patients' needs for access with the physician capacity is a better approach to solving these access issues. It will require a change in the physicians' behavior, which is more likely to occur if they are presented with the right data. This information will also help them to understand the problem better and become actively involved in solving it. They may decide to change how they schedule patients, as illustrated in Exhibit 6.2. In this case, Dr. Atkinson agreed to have open slots for same-day appointments in ten-minute time periods for the last hour of each half-day. Dr. Brighton agreed to schedule more time for physicals and routine or follow-up visits. These changes resulted in increased access for both physicians.

They may also decide to look at the work the personnel in the office do and determine that having the registered nurse serve as a triage nurse, talking to patients about their concerns and giving them advice on home treatment, would be a better service to the patients. By reducing inappropriate patient visits, more

EXHIBIT 6.2. REVISED SCHEDULE FOR DR. ATKINSON AND DR. BRIGHTON.

Dr. Atkinson			Dr. Brighton		
	Patient Name	Type of Visit		Patient Name	Type of Visit
8:00		New pt. H&P	9:00		Yearly physical
8:15			9:10		
8:30			9:20		
8:45		Routine visit	9:30		Illness
9:00		Routine visit	9:40		Chronic care F/U
9:15		Well child	9:50		
9:30			10:00		Well child exam
9:45		Annual gyn	10:10		
10:00			10:20		Annual gyn
10:15		Follow-up	10:30		
10:30		Yearly physical	10:40		Follow-up
10:45			10:50		Follow-up
11:00			11:00		Illness
11:10		Illness	11:10		Illness
11:20		Illness	11:20		Illness
11:30		Hold for acute	11:30		Hold for acute
11:40		Hold for acute	11:40		Hold for acute
11:50		Hold for acute	11:50		Hold for acute
12:00			12:00		

**EXHIBIT 6.2. REVISED SCHEDULE
FOR DR. ATKINSON AND DR. BRIGHTON.** *(continued)*

1:00		Yearly physical	1:00		Illness
1:15			1:10		Illness
1:30			1:20		Illness
1:45		Chronic care F/U	1:30		Routine visit
2:00		Routine visit	1:40		Follow-up
2:15		Well child exam	1:50		Follow-up
2:30			2:00		Hold for acute
2:45		Chronic care F/U	2:10		Hold for acute
3:00		Chronic care F/U	2:20		Hold for acute
3:15		Illness	2:30		Routine visit
3:30		Illness	2:40		Chronic care F/U
3:45		Illness	2:50		
4:00		Illness	3:00		New pt. physical
4:10		Routine visit	3:10		
4:20			3:20		
4:30		Hold for acute	3:30		
4:40		Hold for acute	3:40		Well child exam
4:50		Hold for acute	3:50		
	Total patients = 26		4:00		Annual gyn
			4:10		
			4:20		Illness
			4:30		Illness
			4:40		Acute
			4:50		Acute
				Total patients = 31	

access can be made available for those who need to be seen. Hiring another physician as the only solution could be an expensive and probably unnecessary alternative and might not solve the perception of access held by the patients of these two physicians.

Understanding Technology

Computers are essential for storing and presenting data, so having an understanding of the computer systems from which the data come is very important. In the practice environment it is not unusual for there to be many modules within the computer system that receive and store information differently. Many offices have an information system for registration, patient demographics, scheduling, laboratory and x-ray reporting, billing, and financial analysis of the practice. In fact, some systems have multiple databases in which patient and practice information is stored, some using different hardware platforms and different software programs. The numbers of data reported out of these systems may not match, causing the physicians to perceive a credibility gap. Following is an example of how data entry and reporting can give different views of a physician's work and cause a credibility problem.

A group practice decides to report encounters as a measure in their physician profile. How the data about encounters are obtained will affect the results. Among the ways to look at encounters, one is to use the scheduling system and the other is the billing system. Both track encounters but report them differently.

Suppose Dr. Stevens tends to keep track of patient visits on her own through the scheduling system and keeps a printout of all the patients she has seen on a daily basis. Week by week she sees that she is averaging about one hundred patient visits per week. She has a good idea, month to month, how many patients she has seen. She can account for days she is out of the office and knows she will have lower patient numbers during the months she takes vacation. She feels her data are very accurate. Her data collection reveals the numbers shown in Table 6.4. However, the profile she receives on a monthly basis from administration never seems to correlate with these numbers. Why is that?

The group administrator decided to look at patient encounters based on claims data because of the important link among patient visits, charges, and accounts receivable. Claims data are excellent sources of information about the services patients have received from a practice, but they can add variation to the report depending on which element is looked at. For example, the information on the report will look different if

TABLE 6.4. PATIENT ENCOUNTERS FOR DR. STEVENS FROM THE SCHEDULING SYSTEM.

Dr. Stevens' March Scheduling Data[a]		Patients Seen
Week One	March 1–3	55
Week Two	March 6–10	98
Week Three	March 13–17	102
Week Four	March 20–24[b]	76
Week Five	March 27–31	99
	Total	430

[a]A normal workweek includes nine half-day sessions and Thursday afternoons off.

[b]One day academic leave this week.

the date of service, reflecting the day of the encounter, or the date of posting, reflecting the day the bill was posted, is used in the profile.

Data for the billing system are entered each day through charge capture: each physician fills out a charge slip for each encounter giving a level of service and the diagnosis. In most cases, the physician does this each day, but sometimes there is a delay in this process. The medical encounter slip is routed to the billing clerk, who enters it into the billing system. Most of the patient bills are entered within a few days of the patient visit. Thus, the date entered will be different from the visit or service date for many patients. Also, some of the charges may be entered but reversed later because of errors in insurance information, problems with secondary insurance, changes in the initial charge, or something else. At some point, the bill for each patient visit is finally posted. Depending on all the factors, the posting date can vary weeks or months from the actual date of service.

Table 6.5 presents the encounter report for the physicians during the first quarter, including Dr. Stevens's data. According to the March data, there may be no correlation with actual patients seen during that period. The numbers will include patients Dr. Stevens saw the previous weeks or months and may not include those seen in the last few days of March because of delays in processing.

The point is that if the information sent to the physician about patient encounters within a certain period is based on posted charges and not actual encounters, she will see a discrepancy in the data; consequently, she will not trust the report and instead will trust her own system of hand counting.

Gaining physician trust rests on how the data for feedback are chosen and how closely they correlate to what the physician knows. Involving the physician in the decision about where to obtain the reported data will help credibility. It is also important to explain the details of how the data are obtained for reporting. Once everyone understands where the data come from and how to interpret them, the data will be more useful and accurate.

TABLE 6.5. PATIENT ENCOUNTER REPORT USING POSTED BILLING DATA.

	January	February	March	Year to Date
Dr. Anderson	405	362	423	1,190
Dr. Williams	340	419	302	1,061
Dr. Stevens	378	395	416	1,189
Dr. Miller	412	254	378	1,044
Dr. Chang	388	379	418	1,185
Total	1,923	1,809	1,937	5,669

Presenting Profiling Data

Some of the many tools for presenting data to physicians are simple and easily understood, and others have an academic complexity that makes them difficult to read and interpret. A physician who cannot interpret the report quickly is unlikely to use it. Even worse, misinterpretation of data and basing decisions on that misinterpretation can lead to a lost opportunity for improvement. It can also have serious consequences for individual physicians (Shwayder, 1997).

Here, patient surveys will be used as an example of how information needs to be presented for the physicians to understand fact versus fancy in the data. Patient surveys are one of many available means for measuring and improving patient care and service, and many group practices have begun initiatives to improve patient satisfaction.

Choosing the right tool is clearly important. A good patient satisfaction survey can provide helpful information about areas of improvement that can lead to tremendous differences in patients' overall experiences. Practices choosing to use their own internal survey will require someone with an understanding of survey techniques who knows how to interpret the results.

Most patient satisfaction surveys contain several questions, usually divided into those about the service aspects of their experience and their interpersonal experiences—those with the physicians and providers and those with the support staff. Some surveys devote a few questions to each category and do not provide as much depth as one devoted to asking questions in one particular area. For example, some groups have chosen to try to improve communication between the physicians and the patients, and then use a survey that explores only that area. Some are concerned about patients' experiences with the service and facilities and use surveys that focus on these aspects.

Large, professionally designed patient satisfaction surveys may also allow a group practice to compare itself to others. Benchmarking can be a helpful way to add credibility to the process. However, choosing the right cohorts to be compared to is very important. Tailoring the survey to the needs of the organization is not usually possible in benchmarking. Because of the large number of practices included in the survey, the questions will have to be standardized. Comparing one's group with a large number of similar practices nevertheless can still provide valuable information.

Following are two examples of patient satisfaction surveys and their interpretation.

A large group practice with more than a hundred primary care physicians has been measuring patient satisfaction for each new physician in the practice after one year as part of a performance appraisal process. Over a number of years, the data they have collected allow them to profile their physicians, comparing their new physicians to other new physicians they hired in the past. The patient satisfaction surveys are primarily aimed at looking at physician communication skills. Physicians are compared to their partners in the same department on these skills and to the group practice as a whole. Some departments score very highly with their patients, raising the standard for the whole organization.

Table 6.6 shows an example of the results for Dr. Lindeman, who is in a department that for a variety of reasons generally scores lower in patient satisfaction than other departments. This physician compares favorably with the other physicians within the

TABLE 6.6. PATIENT SATISFACTION SURVEY RESULTS FOR DR. LINDEMAN.

Patient Questions	Department Score	(A)	Physician Score	(B)	All Departments' Scores
Dr. Lindeman					
1. . . . is concerned about my comfort.	2.8		3.0	—	3.9
2. . . . spends enough time with me.	2.6		2.8	—	3.8
3. . . . sits down while talking with me.	2.9		2.9	—	3.7
4. . . . answers my questions respectfully.	3.1		3.2	-	4.0
5. . . . listens to what I am saying.	3.4		3.5	-	4.2
6. . . . explains my condition or diagnosis.	2.8		3.0	-	3.9
7. . . . provides me with results of tests or x-rays.	3.2	+	3.9		3.8
8. . . . explains my lab tests or x-rays.	3.4		3.5	—	4.2
9. . . . explains medications to me.	2.5		2.9	—	3.8
10. . . . provides information to help me make decisions.	2.9		3.1	—	3.9
11. . . . is concerned for me as a person.	3.0	+	3.5	-	4.1
12. . . . refers me to consultants as needed.	3.7		4.0		4.3
13. . . . is sensitive to my needs.	2.9	+	3.2		3.9
14. . . . I am generally pleased with this doctor's care.	3.2		3.5		3.8
15. . . . I would recommend this doctor to a friend	3.3		3.0	—	4.1
Total Scores	45.7		49.0	—	59.4

Note: Column A is a comparison to average scores of doctors in the same department. Column B is a comparison to average scores of doctors in all departments.

Key: + = 1 standard deviation above; ++ = 2 standard deviations above; - = 1 standard deviation below; — = 2 standard deviations below.

department but not to the group as a whole. An alternative way to present the data for Dr. Lindeman is in a graphical form, which emphasizes these differences (see Figure 6.1).

If Dr. Lindeman were to receive only department-specific data, he may get a false sense of having at least average communication skills and may see no need to improve. His patients, however, are giving him feedback to suggest that he scores significantly below other physicians in this large group practice. In this case, the organization may want to spend some time and effort to improve the skills of all the physicians in this department, thus increasing patient satisfaction overall.

The second example is of data that a practice may receive from a benchmarking study.

In this survey group practices are compared to other similar practices across the country. One large group practice that chose to use this survey includes many offices consisting of two to five physicians per office. Patients who are chosen randomly from

FIGURE 6.1. GRAPHICAL DISPLAY OF PATIENT SATISFACTION SURVEY RESULTS FOR DR. LINDEMAN.

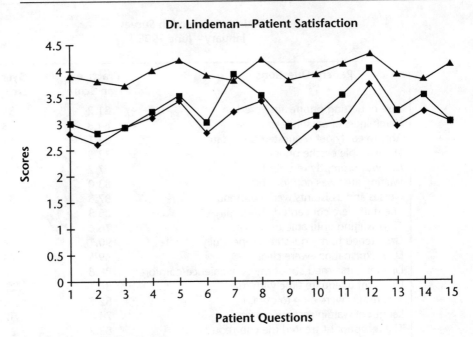

♦ Department Score
■ Dr. Lindeman
▲ All Departments' Score

the schedules are asked to rate their experience on a scale of 1 (poor) to 5 (excellent). The surveys are sent out on a continuous basis throughout the year, and the results are reported quarterly. The response rate varies for each practice, and therefore the denominator varies among the groups. A total score is presented for each category.

One group's scores range from 70 to 90 on a range of 0 to 100 total points. The report is presented in Figure 6.2.

On initial glance, an overall score of 83 may look good, but the important comparison is to see what percentile that places the practice in when compared to the other practices in the survey. As is turns out, a score of 83 in this case places this group in the thirty-second percentile overall, not as good as initially thought.

Patient motivation is an important determinant to how accurate the survey data are. Patients who are loyal and devoted to a particular physician practice are more likely to respond to a questionnaire sent to them from their provider. These patients as a rule are more satisfied with their care than those who may

FIGURE 6.2. REPORT OF PATIENT SATISFACTION SURVEY.

Patient Satisfaction Survey
January – June 1998

Patient Questions	Practice Mean Score	Overall Percentile
Ease of getting phone answered	81.2	35
Helpfulness of person taking call	84.8	48
Able to easily get requested time/date	83.1	62
Dr. available on the phone	73.5	11
Call was promptly returned	77.2	22
Waiting area was comfortable	83.0	19
Nurses and assistants were courteous	87.3	30
The staff were concerned about me	85.3	31
Time waiting until able to see Dr.	76.6	29
Dr. listened to my questions repectfully	90.1	26
Dr.'s explanations were clear	89.5	24
Dr. was concerned about my convenience/comfort	88.8	27
Dr. spent adequate time with me	86.1	25
Test results were easy to obtain	82.7	54
Length of wait in reception area	74.8	37
The receptionist treated me courteously	83.7	37
Average for all questions	83	32

FIGURE 6.2. REPORT OF PATIENT SATISFACTION SURVEY. *(continued)*

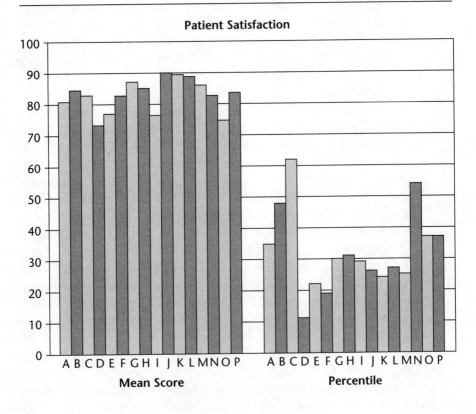

Patient Satisfaction

Mean Score

Percentile

A   Ease of getting phone answered
B   Helpfulness of person taking call
C   Able to easily get requested time/date
D   Dr. available on the phone
E   Call was promptly returned
F   Waiting area was comfortable
G   Nurses and assistants were courteous
H   The staff were concerned about me
I   Time waiting until able to see Dr.
J   Dr. listened to my questions repectfully
K   Dr.'s explanations were clear
L   Dr. was concerned about my convenience/comfort
M   Dr. spent adequate time with me
N   Test results were easy to obtain
O   Length of wait in reception area
P   The receptionist treated me courteously

choose to dispose of the survey as a nuisance, especially if they have already decided to leave a practice. If this assumption is true, then fairly high scores should be expected. Scores of 2 percent poor, 5 percent fair, 23 percent good, 50 percent very good, and 20 percent excellent are probably not good scores. Ideally, one would want to have all of the responses falling into the last two categories, with a predominance in the excellent category.

In the example survey, on the question regarding, "Does you doctor listen to your questions respectfully?" a score of 90.1 may seem very high. In comparison to all the other practices in the survey, however, this practice ranks only in the twenty-sixth percentile—not very good. It is important to include an explanation of the data to the physicians so that the profile makes sense. Sharing only the data that represent the score to the physicians, and not the percentile rank, may not allow appropriate interpretation. They may think a raw score of 83 represents 83 percent, which is incorrect. In this case, a score of 83 places this group in the thirty-second percentile overall.

When presenting data to physicians, it is very important to consider how they will interpret what is given to them. A face-to-face meeting is the best way to provide feedback to a physician, especially on sensitive material like patient satisfaction. Time-consuming as it can be, a meeting offers the best opportunity to explain what the data mean. If a meeting is not feasible, then complete explanations should be included with the data, so that the physicians will understand what they are seeing. The profiling staff should be available to answer any questions physicians may have about the data and must be prepared to explain how the information was obtained and the analysis that was used. Kibbe (1996) advises that "physicians must first understand the key information management methods associated with physician profiling and know what questions to ask of those producing profiles."

Effect of Measurement on Physician Behavior

It has been well documented that the very act of measuring someone's behavior begins to change it. This Hawthorne effect seems to be particularly true when looking at patient care issues.

One of the best examples comes from a study at Park Nicollet Clinic in Minnesota, which initiated a study several years ago that looked at mammography rates for all physicians who treat women over age fifty. Specialists outside primary care were included because several of them did primary care for their specialty patients. By feeding back the information to the physicians each year, along with the recommendation that women over age fifty have a yearly mammogram, it was found that more patients had received a mammogram than in the previous year. Physicians were given a simple graph like the one in Figure 6.3 that reflected the percentage of women who had received a mammogram in their practice. Each physician knew which point on the graph represented him or her. They could see how their colleagues did but could not identify individual colleagues by the data on the graph. The physicians knew they would be measured each year. Virtually all physicians improved their rates. By the fifth year of the study, it was no longer necessary to measure their work, because the physicians had incorporated ordering the mammograms into their routine care. It may be of interest to note that this change occurred with *no* financial incentive to change.

Because it is possible to change physician behavior with good information that is presented in an easy-to-understand fashion, determining what to measure is an important decision. In a sense, when clinics choose to measure something, they have made a value judgment that this area is important enough to the organization or individual to measure it. Here is an example of what can happen when a measure is chosen without thinking about the effect it may have on the practice over time.

A six-physician primary care practice has been growing as managed care contracts bring new patients. Some of their physicians' fee-for-service patients have changed to the same managed care plans. Managed care is new to them, and they are eager to become involved because it is an opportunity for their practice to grow. The physicians have agreed to receive equal base salaries based on market surveys plus an incentive based on productivity.

The practice manager and the physicians decide to measure physician productivity by number of encounters and charges over time. The manager shares these data with the physicians so that they can see how they compare with their partners. Over time, she notices that the number of patient visits per physician are increasing. Some physicians have instructed their staff to keep their schedules full and to shorten the visit times. The staff are very busy seeing these additional patients and are working overtime.

The manager follows the coding profiles and now notices that the physicians are coding at higher levels than previously. This could be appropriate, since they have been taught the proper coding and documentation procedures. Still, the practice manager becomes concerned because the increased patient visits are partly due to an increase in the total number of visits per year for each patient. The capitation was based on an assumed 3.5 patient visits per year, but in actuality the practice is seeing patients on average 4.5 times per year. This is true for all patients since the physicians treat their managed care patients the same as their fee-for-service patients. Collections on the fee-for-service patients have also been discounted over this time from 82 percent of gross charges to 77 percent on average. According to the physician profiles, it appears that they have all increased their productivity because of increasing numbers of patient visits and charges.

Productivity, as measured by total individual patients seen and practice revenues, may not have gone up to the extent that the number of encounters and charges would

FIGURE 6.3. PERCENTAGE OF WOMEN WHO RECEIVED AN ANNUAL MAMMOGRAM, PARK NICOLLET CLINIC.

Percent	1987	1988	1989	1990
100	OO		O	OO
98				
96				O
94		O	OOO	OOOOOOO
92	O	O	OO	OOOOOOOOO
90		OOOOOO	OO	OOOOOX
88	O	OOOO	OOOOOOOOOO	OO
86	OO	OOOO	OOOX	O
84	OO	OO	OOO	O
82	OOO	OOOX	OO	OOO
80	OOOOOO	OOOOO	OO	OOO
78	OO	OOO	OO	O
76	O	O	OOOO	OO
74	X		O	
72		OO		
70	OOO	O	O	OO
68	O	O	O	
66	OOO			
64	O	O	OO	O
62	OO	O		
60				
58				O
56			O	
54	O			
52				
50	O	O		
48				
46				
44				
42	O			
40	O			
38				
36				
34				
32	O			
30				
28				

Note: O = individual physician; X = average percentage

suggest. The costs of providing care to these increasing patient volumes have gone up due to staff overtime pay at the same time that revenues are being discounted or fixed. Paying physicians an incentive based solely on charges (not revenues) and encounters has resulted in an incentive payment that exceeds what the practice can support.

How does a practice choose the elements of the profile that measure true physician productivity? In a mixed fee-for-service and capitated practice, what are the profile elements that represent productivity? Higher productivity in the fee-for-service environment means more visits, more tests, and more procedures. In a managed care setting it means fewer visits, tests, and procedures. Perhaps a better measurement would be the total number of individual patients served *and* total revenue compared to costs for each visit. Choosing to measure physicians this way, and basing the incentive on this profile, may lead the physicians to change their practice styles to be more conscious of costs related to patient care and the decreasing dollars available to provide it. Over time their practice profile will change as they find better, more efficient ways of caring for patients and serving their health needs.

Conclusion

Profiling of physician group practices begins with an understanding of the system of care in which they work—both the work involved in the processes of patient care and the work of all the individuals who participate in the care team. The information must reflect actual work in order for physicians to respect and want to use it. Involving physicians and other health care professionals in helping to decide what is worth measuring and what is not is important.

The elements of measurement must be a true representation of the physician work. Because they come from a computer does not mean that this is the best measurement. It is important to understand how the data were entered and reported. Running a pilot profile and having physicians compare what the report shows with what they know is a useful exercise. If there are too many inconsistencies, the practice may have to search for another data source. In addition, it is important to check the initial assumptions about each selected data element.

Data must be presented to physicians in an easily interpretable and useful format; complicated data presentations that require a lot of time and effort to interpret may not be helpful to them. On the other hand, being too simplistic can be problematic. Misinterpretation may be avoided by being available to explain the profiling information. If there are consistent complaints about the presentation format of the data, profiling administrators should be open to changing it into a more useful format.

The decision to select a particular physician performance measurement will most likely change physician behavior. This can be beneficial if the selection is aligned with an overall practice goal. However, measuring physician performance on elements that are not supportive of a practice's values and core business may lead to a negative effect on the organization as a whole. Doctors will want to score well on whatever profile element is chosen. Thus, administrators must use caution and involve the leadership in deciding what is the best information to profile and feed back to physicians. It is one of the best ways to influence physicians to align their personal goals with the goals of the organization and the needs of their patients.

Finally, exhibit care when trying to profile: remember that fancy can creep into the process.

References

Bell, K. M. "Physician Profiling: 12 Critical Points." *Journal of Ambulatory Care Management,* 1996, *19*(1), 81–85.

Kibbe, D. C. "Is Your Performance Profile Accurate?" *Family Practice Management,* 1996, *3*(8), 68–75.

Micklitsch, C. N., and Ryan-Mitlyng, T. A. *Physician Performance Management: Tool for Survival and Success.* Englewood, Colo.: MGMA, 1995.

Rosenstein, A. H. "Provider Profiling: Promises and Pitfalls." *Managed Care Medicine,* Oct. 1995, pp. 10–12, 32–35.

Ruffin, M., "Physician Profiling: Trends and Implications." [http://tii.ruffin.com/v0000133.htm]. Nov. 1995.

Shwayder, J. M. "They're Not Calling Me an Outlier Anymore." *Medical Economics,* 1997, *74*(10), 87–88, 91–92.

Solberg, L. I., Mosser, G., and McDonald, S. "The Three Faces of Performance Measurement: Improvement, Accountability, and Research." *Journal on Quality Improvement,* 1997, *23*(3), 135–147.

CHAPTER SEVEN

PROFILING DATA TO DETERMINE PHYSICIAN COMPENSATION

Anne Sales, Jay Noren, Douglas A. Conrad, Jim Tufano

An organization that is determining compensation for physicians both employs the physicians in some meaningful sense (they are not treated as independent contractors or consultants) and retains control of some or all of the administrative and clinical records used in treating patients. This means that the organization is expected to be able to produce data for each provider that is more detailed and, it is hoped, more reliable than the types of data used for purely administrative claims submitted to a third-party payer. This chapter will not address models that practices use to decide how to distribute or allocate revenues (Levine, 1996). It assumes that those decisions have been made and the issue now is how to allocate compensation to individuals on a relatively rational and equitable basis.

Selecting Elements of a Profiling System

One of the most common uses of profiling, but also one of the most controversial, is to determine compensation for providers. Profiling systems can assist managers in administering fair, reasonable, and justifiable compensation systems, but the systems must be viewed as acceptable by the participants in order to be accepted.

Elements of provider profiles used for compensation must be aligned with the strategic goals of the organization. It is particularly important to ensure that elements are essential to the goals and mission of the organization for two reasons.

First, the ability to demonstrate how the elements of a profiling system used to determine compensation are integrated with strategic goals assists physicians and other providers in understanding how those elements were selected. Second, there is a greater likelihood that the profiling system will stay focused and streamlined. There is a temptation to select profiling elements, particularly for compensation purposes, that other groups use in an effort to legitimize their use by referring to others using them. Nevertheless, each organization should ask itself how each element fits into its organizational design, strategies, and goals. For example, a medical group composed largely of procedurally oriented specialists may choose to include elements related to number and quality of procedures, while one focused mostly on primary care may choose to focus instead on patient visits and compliance with preventive care guidelines.

Elements used for compensation determination must be measurable and relatively objective. Reliance on subjective elements is likely to result in conflict over the use of these elements in determining compensation. The bottom line is that if effort is put into selecting the elements of the system carefully at the outset, less work will need to be done to convince providers of the fairness and appropriateness of the system when it is applied to them.

Elements must be applicable to the individual provider level. The measurement must be attributable to the individual rather than to a group level such as a clinic or team, unless the individual is being evaluated as part of a team. Data elements used in determining compensation must vary by individuals.

Finally, it is essential to assess data on all three axes of the health care triangle: cost, quality, and access. Although it is tempting to focus on cost in compensation models, an exclusive focus on cost makes it easier for providers to game the compensation system by focusing their efforts on lowering costs, sometimes without appropriate concern for quality of care or the effects on access to care.

Data Related to Cost and Revenue

Cost data are often the easiest to identify as elements of profiling systems related to compensation. High volume, high revenue-generating providers are often those regarded as most valued in an organization, for good reason. Highly productive providers who do not demonstrate high utilization patterns (using resources that cost the organization revenue) often contribute in ways that are easily measured to the bottom line of the organization. These measures alone may produce a skewed profile of a provider's contribution, but they are extremely important in determining how valuable someone's contribution is to the organization.

Utilization Data. Selecting relevant measures is critical to the success of the profiling system. One of the first steps is to decide on measures that reflect the type of workload that best represents the organization or the subunit of the organization included in the profiling system. Office-based or inpatient-based (such as hospitalist) practices typically use encounters or patient contacts as the units to be measured, while procedure-based practices such as surgical services might use procedures as the measure. Whatever measure is used should be easily obtained through electronic data rather than relying on self-reports or requiring hours of labor to extract the data manually from paper-based records. If the organization is not yet at a point where data are retrievable electronically, then systematic profiling for purposes of compensation is probably not appropriate. It is difficult to imagine a profiling system that is used to determine compensation that would not include some type of measure of workload or productivity as one of the fundamental elements.

Although this is a critical element, there are some issues to keep in mind in deciding whether the data available are adequate. One is that utilization measures are always subject to errors in coding. The definitions used in deciding, for example, what a "visit" is are critical, and they must be applied in the same way to all providers. Consider the measure "number of visits per enrolled patient," which is designed to assess one dimension of productivity for an individual provider. Dr. A includes reading electrocardiograms (EKGs) as "visits" because of the way he or his staff code them; he performs this activity several times daily, spending from one to five minutes per EKG. Dr. B's "visits" never include EKG readings, although she does them as frequently as Dr. A does. Her "visits" include only direct face-to-face patient encounters, typically during a clinic visit that lasts from five to fifty minutes. Not surprisingly, Dr. A always has a higher proportion of "visits per enrolled patient" than does Dr. B. Due to the differences in coding (driven by the different definitions used), this measure provides a poor comparison between these two providers.

Most coding-related issues are not this extreme or this obvious. Typically they are not as systematic, but still occur often enough that it is essential to have a plan to check the validity and reliability of the data being used in order to ensure that the profiling system is treating each provider fairly.

Another issue is whether to use the count—such as "number of visits"—as the measure included in the profile or to use a rate, such as "number of visits per enrolled patient." Although it is much easier to use the count than the rate, it does not provide a very fair comparison among providers who work part time compared with those who work full time. The absolute number of visits will be lower for a part-time employee, and the rate, divided by the number of patients being cared for, will probably be more alike for the two providers. The major drawback to using rates rather than counts is that it is not always easy to decide on an appropriate denominator—and the denominator is critical. It must validly represent some population that the provider can legitimately be held accountable for. In this respect, the push toward managed care and care of populations helps to provide the kinds of numbers necessary for denominators. It is becoming standard practice to identify panels of patients enrolled to a particular provider. For primary care providers, this is a reasonable denominator to use for many rates, not just utilization. Finding the equivalent denominator for specialists may not be as simple, but some type of population could be associated with each specialist provider. For example, the panels of the primary care providers referring to that specialist could be combined to form a panel for the specialist.

Cost Data. A related approach is to use a dollar-denominated measure either instead of or in addition to utilization measures. These include gross charges attributable to the provider or some other measure that assigns a dollar value to the work that provider does. As with utilization data, it is necessary to decide how to adjust for providers who work different amounts of time; comparing a full-time clinician's gross charges with those of a provider who is funded 50 percent time to do research would not be a valid comparison without adjusting it by creating a rate of some sort. It might be appropriate to evaluate everyone as a full-time equivalent by extrapolating (for those who do not work full time) from the proportion of time they work to what they might be producing if they were working full time. Although this is appealing as a relatively easy way to adjust for the proportion of a person's time spent working, it requires some assumptions to be made about what would be observed if people were to work more than they do. It might be reasonable to assume that they would, for example, produce double the output (in this case, gross charges) working full time than they produce working half time. This may be a reasonable or, depending on the type of work, invalid assumption. In some cases, the amount of additional work produced for every additional hour worked might actually decline, as in the case of someone whose peak efficiency occurs with a thirty-hour workweek. After that, each additional hour worked might produce diminishing output. This might be the case for clinicians who have psychically intense interactions with their patients, such as psychiatrists doing psychotherapy or a procedurally oriented physician, such as an invasive cardiologist who performs a certain number of procedures per day while working part time. If that cardiologist were to work full time, it is possible that she might perform more procedures than expected if one extrapolated in a straight line, largely because her referral base might grow for a number of reasons. Rather than extrapolating to full time, an alternative is to use an approach that divides gross charges by the number of patients in a panel.

Another concern to bear in mind regarding cost data for profiling is the possibility that because of differences among patient groups in what the practice can charge for services, there are differences in charges attributable to providers that do not really reflect differences in productivity. For example, if patient A is a member of a group that has a discounted fee-for-service rate and patient B is a member of a group with a capitated monthly payment, the actual revenues attributable to a provider who cares for both patients and provides the same service will not be the same. Unless this is adjusted so that the attributable charges for each patient are the same, which might require creating pseudo-bills or some other mechanism, the provider does not get the same credit for both patients. Although this may adjust itself for each provider, a provider who happens to have more patients from a group with a highly discounted rate or one who has more capitated patients may look considerably less productive on gross charges than someone who has more patients with a less discounted rate. Although these providers do in fact produce different amounts of revenue for the organization, this difference is probably not under their control. A compensation system that does not adjust for this kind of externally controlled difference is likely to be perceived as unfair.

The Other Side of Utilization and Cost. This discussion has focused on using utilization and cost data to measure a provider's positive contribution to the organization. The other side of cost and utilization measures relevant to profiling for compensation is the degree to which provider practice patterns may indicate potential excess cost to the organization. This is particularly relevant in today's market, where an ever-increasing proportion of patients in a practice receive services under some kind of capitated arrangement. Examples of this kind of utilization include laboratory and other diagnostic charges, prescribing patterns (if the practice bears the cost of prescriptions through a capitation payment), or, in some cases, return visits that may be unnecessary or could be delegated to a lower-cost provider. The type of payment (whether capitation or not) will have an important effect on which types of charges should be included in a profiling system.

Many of the issues with regard to ensuring comparability of effort (such as time worked) are relevant in considering data elements of this type. Another consideration is the correct attribution of charges or costs to the appropriate provider. It is not unusual for a primary care provider to refer a patient to a specialist and have diagnostic charges incurred by the specialist. If the primary care provider is being profiled on laboratory or diagnostic test utilization or charges incurred by another provider, those charges should not be attributed to the primary care provider unless he or she has sufficient authority to control the costs.

A final component of cost and utilization data is the degree to which they reflect access or availability of care. Utilization in particular reflects capacity as well as cost. Capacity determines access. This is a difficult area because there are few standards that are based on empirical evidence that can be used to make decisions about what constitutes the "right" number of patients who can safely be cared for by, for example, a primary care provider. In many respects, answers to these kinds of questions reflect judgments based on experience and, to some extent, anecdotal evidence. However, it is still important to include some measures directly related to access in a profiling system—for example, waiting time for new patient appointments, waiting time for follow-up appointments, waiting time for referrals to specialty consultations, and waiting time in the clinic after a patient checks in. The measure chosen should reflect the kinds of work that are most important to the practice or indicate improvement in areas that have been problems in the past.

Measures Related to Quality of Care

There is a very large literature on quality of care in both inpatient and outpatient settings. Many of these measures have been tested for use in health plan report cards and other large-scale systems for monitoring quality of care.

Aside from issues of data quality (discussed in Chapters Two and Three), the biggest problem in applying measures related to quality of care to individual providers is that often an individual provider has only a limited number of patients to whom a measure applies. An example is measuring appropriate mammogram use in a provider's panel. Even with a large panel (one thousand or more active patients), there might only be a relatively small number of women meeting guidelines for screening mammography (relatively small in this instance would be anything under one hundred patients). Any time that there are small numbers in both the potential numerator and denominator on a measure, such as "appropriate use of screening mammography," the potential for finding rates that are due more to random chance than to observable reality is fairly high. Few of the quality measures apply to an entire panel of primary care patients, after excluding patients for whom a service might not be appropriate, so that issues of small number affect most of the measures in this area. This problem is usually compounded by the need to sample patients to retrieve data, which often requires manual chart audit. In this case, the numbers (not very large even if the entire panel were being included) become even smaller, leading to a still greater problem. Small differences among providers can seem much greater than they really are because of sampling issues and chance variation that do not reflect true differences in quality of care. One way to compensate partially for the problem of small numbers is to accumulate observations over time (for example, sampling 5 to 10 percent of relevant charts each month and accumulating six months' worth of observations before including the findings in the profiling system).

It is tempting to ask whether it is really necessary to include these measures in a compensation system, given the inherent difficulties, and many organizations do not. Nevertheless, it is important to think through the potential consequences of omitting these measures. If a profiling system does not include measures of quality of care, there is a risk that providers will adjust their effort to improve, say, a laboratory test measure in their profile. This could result in limiting laboratory testing for patients; if no measures reflecting quality of care (based on guidelines or other accepted protocols) are included in the profiling system, patients might not receive the diagnostic tests they need. This could be considered gaming the profiling system; it reflects a rational, if not entirely ethical, response on the part of individual providers to the incentives they perceive to be operating. Measures of quality of care included in the profiling system should be geared toward reducing the likelihood of this kind of response.

Issues of Adjustment

An essential component in comparing all of these kinds of data across providers is to attempt to adjust for differences among patients attributable to their underlying health status. Bell (1996) points to the controversy about whether adjustment should be made for both health status and the patient's likelihood of seeking treatment in a profiling system, but in either case, some level of case mix adjustment must be made.

There are a number of approaches to making such an adjustment. One of the more popular relies on the diagnostic code used to describe the primary presenting problem for each visit or encounter. These Ambulatory Care Groupings (ACGs) (Tucker, Weiner, Honigfeld, and Parton, 1996) have been shown to work relatively well for many measures of utilization in the ambulatory setting. Other outpatient case mix adjustment approaches include the Chronic Disease Score (Clark and others, 1995), which uses pharmacy data to adjust for underlying health status, and other diagnosis-based systems described by Ellis, Pope, and Iezzoni (1996). Inpatient measures (probably mostly applicable to specialists, rather than primary care physicians) can be adjusted for case mix using a variety of measures adapted to the inpatient setting (see Iezzoni, 1997, for examples).

Choosing case mix adjustment strategies requires some willingness to invest time in testing strategies and deciding which is most appropriate for the type of measure being used for compensation profiling. It may require contracting for expert assistance to decide how best to achieve case mix adjustment for the set of measures used in the profiling system, and different measures may require different adjusters. For example, an organization may choose to include inpatient days of care in the profile for providers whose practices are largely outpatient based. It is important to think through the question of whether to treat this as an outpatient or an inpatient measure, depending on the types of patient population being cared for. If a health care provider thinks that it reflects characteristics of an outpatient population, it may want to use an ambulatory case mix adjustment strategy. If it appears instead to be an inpatient measure, then inpatient-based methods of adjusting, often based on diagnosis-related groups, may be more appropriate. (Case mix adjustment is discussed in further detail in Chapter Five.)

Data Validity

Much of the problem of small numbers reflects the relatively small numbers in the panels of patients enrolled to individual providers. Determining appropriate panel size is not an easy issue, although ultimately panel size is one of the most important forces driving provider effort and the level of compensation that should reward that effort. One way is to aggregate observations over time to try to adjust for small numbers. Another approach is to consider the processes of producing the care being delivered to patients, which is reflected in the elements of the profiling system. Many of these care processes involve teams rather than individual providers, and the teams may include more than one clinical provider, as well as ancillary staff who provide or assist in providing those services. It may be appropriate to include an entire team in some measures rather than focusing on the individual provider. The trade-off may be in terms of complexity of the system, compared to a simpler but potentially less valid (and possibly less fair) system that attributes services to one individual rather than to the team that produces them. This is a decision that needs to be made at the organizational level and depends in large part on the type of organization and its culture (Micklitsch and Ryan-Mitlyng, 1996).

Trends in Physician Compensation Methods

During the past decade physician compensation methods have evolved substantially, particularly in managed care organizations and large group practices. These trends underscore the need for increasingly sophisticated physician profiling methods for compensation based on multiple measures of cost, quality, and access. Since 1987 the Medical Group Management Association (MGMA) has surveyed member practices on physician compensation and production. The most recent survey, conducted in 1997, solicited data from all 5,725 MGMA member group practices; 1,675 practices responded (29 percent response rate), comprising 35,254 providers (MGMA, 1998). The survey measured productivity using five components: gross charges, ambulatory encounters, hospital encounters, surgical/anesthesia cases, and Resource-Based Relative-Value Scale units provided. MGMA results during the past five years reflect the volatility of compensation trends and demonstrate the need for accurate physician profiling methods. Trends in total compensation, primary versus specialty physicians, and managed care differentials merit attention. The period 1992 to 1996 saw steadily decreasing annual rates of increase in median compensation, from 6.8 percent to 0.9 percent providers (MGMA, 1997). Particularly noteworthy was the difference in five-year change (1993–1997) for primary care physicians (general internal medicine, general pediatrics, family medicine), which was higher than that for specialists (9.26 percent versus 6.34 percent) (MGMA, 1998). This trend is illustrated in Table 7.1, which compares the differences between primary care physicians and specialists in various managed care environments. The compensation for primary care physicians increased 2 percent for high-managed-care environments, whereas for specialists, the compensation decreased 11 percent under the same conditions. Despite these trends, specialty median compensation continues to exceed primary care substantially (by 62 percent—$220,476 versus $135,791 in the 1997 survey).

Analysis of the most recent three years of MGMA surveys indicates increasing compensation volatility. Based on the 1994 survey, Conrad and others described four broad categories of individual physician compensation: (1) fee-for-service or production based, (2) salary, (3) group-based equal shares, and (4) capitation. In 1994 the predominant form was pure fee-for-service/production based (35 percent for primary care physicians and 34 percent for specialists). Base salary plus incentive ranked second (23 percent for primary care physicians and 20 percent for specialists). The incentives in this method take various forms, including patient service volume (similar to fee-for-service methods), patient satisfaction measures, cost-containment success, quality of care, and organizational or community services contributions. Third ranking were methods employing a majority of fee-for-service combined with other modes (21 percent for primary care physicians and 19 percent for specialists). Note that combining pure fee-for-service and majority fee-for-service demonstrates the overall dominance of fee-for-service at 56 percent for primary care physicians and 53 percent for specialists. Pure salary follows fourth in ranking (14 percent for primary care physicians and 12 percent for specialists). Group members' equal shares and capitation combined contribute a very small

TABLE 7.1. GROUP PRACTICES PHYSICIAN COMPENSATION, 1994 AND 1996.

Percentage Managed Care	Primary Care	Specialists
No managed care	$138,260	$203,225
10 percent or less	$136,700	$248,970
11–50 percent	$135,000	$231,422
51–100 percent	$140,914	$184,502

proportion in comparison: 2 percent for primary care physicians and 7 percent for specialists for equal shares and 5 percent for primary care physicians and 8 percent for specialists for capitation. Comparison of these results to the 1997 survey (the most recent one) indicates a shift from pure (100 percent) fee-for-service/production based emphasis toward a greater emphasis on mixed salary and fee-for-service/production. Table 7.2 summarizes these trends.

The increasing use of financial incentives for physicians in managed care organizations intensifies the need for improved physician profiling methods for compensation purposes. For example, U.S. Healthcare, a managed care organization, pays cash bonuses based on Health Plan Employer Data and Information Set (HEDIS) performance data and other measures created by the organization, including report cards to individual physicians addressing efficiency, effectiveness, and patient satisfaction. U.S. Healthcare uses member surveys sent to 1.5 million enrollees yearly (with a 30 to 38 percent response rate) as a basis for patient satisfaction measures. The method employs five components in quality-of-care measures: (1) access through reduction in geographic or demographic barriers, (2) appropriateness of care, (3) disease-specific process of care, (4) outcomes assessed

TABLE 7.2. GROUP PRACTICES' COMPENSATION METHODOLOGY, 1994 AND 1997.

Method	Percentage of Groups Using This Method for Primary Care Physicians		Percentage of Groups Using This Method for Specialist Physicians	
	1994	1997	1994	1997
100 percent fee-for-service/production based	35	29	34	30
50–99 percent fee-for-service/production based (remainder some other method)	21	22	19	20
50–99 percent guaranteed salary (remainder incentive)	23	22	20	18
100 percent straight salary	14	19	12	12
100 percent group member equal shares	2	1	7	9
Capitation and other	5	7	8	10
Total	100	100	100	99

Sources: Conrad and others (1996); MGMA (1997).

by patient's functional status at six, twelve, and eighteen months postservice, and (5) patient satisfaction documentation (Appleby, 1995). Using these methods in 1994, the company distributed $2.2 million cash bonuses to obstetricians/gynecologists ranked in the top twenty-fifth percentile in reduced cesarean section rates (Appleby, 1995; Hanchak, 1997).

Of course, such approaches do not avoid criticism. The criticism of incentives focuses primarily on the questionable meaningfulness or accuracy of quality measures. Nonetheless, the use of incentives appears increasingly with the models varying by organization. The Kaiser method, unlike that of U.S. Healthcare, does not employ direct cash incentives but considers performance measures in periodic pay raises. Principal Kaiser measures address technical quality of care, member satisfaction, and utilization (Appleby, 1995).

Clearly there exists much demand for valid performance measures for physician compensation decisions, particularly in managed care organizations. The need for further development of physician-profiling methods will continue to increase.

Conclusion

Profiling for compensation is a highly charged, complex process that should consider data on all three axes of the health care triangle: cost, quality, and access. Legitimating the process is very important, and one of the ways many people seek to legitimate the process is to produce complex, intricate systems designed to rationalize as much of the system as possible. It is tempting to search for these kinds of solutions to what are essentially political problems, but engaging in this kind of hyperrationalization can clutter the organization's system. Trying to cover every base and deal with every potential issue also leads to complexity and difficulty. Each measure added to the system increases the cost of constructing and using the system. Each measure added also increases the degree to which the system is open to attack by unhappy providers who feel that the system does not adequately measure their input. Too narrow a system (with only a few measures) will make people feel that they are not being judged fairly. Too wide a system (with a great many measures) will make people feel that they are being intensely scrutinized and open opportunities for disagreement about details rather than the core of someone's performance.

Deciding where to draw the line on how detailed and complex a profiling system should be is essentially a management decision based on judgment and expert knowledge of the organization, as well as a decision subject to political negotiation. However, it is important to align the selected data elements with the strategic goals of the organization. For many organizations, the primary appeal of a profiling system to be used in determining compensation is to reduce the degree to which compensation systems are a political process. It is essential to understand that introducing such a system does not eliminate the political nature of the process. Done well, it should be able to reduce significantly the political aspects of determining compensation.

References

Appleby C. "The Measure of Medical Services." *Hospitals and Health Networks,* June 20, 1995, pp. 26–34.

Bell, K. M. "Physician Profiling: 12 Critical Points." *Journal of Ambulatory Care Management,* 1996, *19*(1), 81–85.

Clark, D. O., and others. "A Chronic Disease Score with Empirically Derived Weights." *Medical Care,* 1995, *33*(8), 783–795.

Conrad, D. A., and others. "Physician Compensation Models in Medical Group Practices." *Journal of Ambulatory Care Management,* 1996, *19*(4), 18–27.

Ellis, R. P., Pope, G. C., and Iezzoni, L. "Diagnosis-Based Risk Adjustment for Medicare Capitation Payments." *Health Care Financing Review,* 1996, *17*(3), 101–128.

Hanchak, N. "A Performance-Based Compensation Model for Obstetricians/Gynecologists." *Clinical Obstetrics and Gynecology,* 1997, *40*(2), 437–445.

Iezzoni, L. I. (ed.). *Risk Adjustment for Measuring Health Care Outcomes.* (2nd ed.). Chicago: Health Administration Press, 1997.

Levine, J. "Compensation Models and Issues for Multispecialty Group Practice." *Journal of Ambulatory Care Management,* 1996, *19*(3), 50–59.

Medical Group Management Association. *Physician Compensation and Production Survey.* Englewood, Colo.: MGMA, 1997.

Medical Group Management Association. *Physician Compensation and Production Survey.* Englewood, Colo.: MGMA, 1998.

Micklitsch, C. N., and Ryan-Mitlyng, T. A. *Physician Performance Management: Tool for Survival and Success.* Englewood, Colo.: Medical Group Management Association, 1996.

Tucker, A. M., Weiner, J. P., Honigfeld, S., and Parton, R. A. "Profiling Primary Care Physician Resource Use: Examining the Application of Case Mix Adjustment." *Journal of Ambulatory Care Management,* 1996, *19*(1), 60–80.

CHAPTER EIGHT

PATIENT SATISFACTION AND PHYSICIAN PROFILING

Philip L. Cyr, Daniel W. Malloy

The U.S. health care system has undergone dramatic changes since the mid-1980s. In addition to providing quality medical care, physicians and their staff are having to adapt to the rapidly evolving business of health care. We have witnessed a substantial growth in the development and utilization of new medical technologies that have shifted a vast portion of medical care from an inpatient to an outpatient setting (Williams and Torrens, 1993), experienced changes in reimbursement mechanisms that emphasize capitated reimbursement arrangements over fee-for-service arrangements, and seen active involvement of large businesses in the form of regional business coalitions (Cronin, 1994). The primary concern of these coalitions is that their employees get the most for every dollar the business allocates toward health care. Therefore, businesses and business coalitions are a major force behind the use of satisfaction data as a form of consumer protection. Together these changes have created a system that uses a population approach to examining the effectiveness of care and has become more consumer conscious. An example of this focus is represented by the question frequently asked by consumers: "Are one health plan's or physician group's patients more satisfied with the care they receive than another's?"

Patient satisfaction has become an important quality of care outcome measure as the examination of our health care system has become population based and more consumer driven. Health plans and group practices commonly use satisfaction ratings to profile physicians and impose financial incentives based on their findings. As a result, it is essential for physicians and health care administrators to have a working knowledge of the measurement and use of patient satisfaction data.

Origins of Patient Satisfaction Measurement

Health care providers and regulators now recognize patient satisfaction as a legitimate measure of health care quality (Ross, Steward, and Sinacore, 1995). This has not always been the case. The use of patient satisfaction as a proxy for health care quality had its origins in the 1960s with the RAND Health Insurance Experiment, which measured the effect that different co-insurance rates had on health care utilization, functional status, and patient satisfaction. Data from this experiment clearly demonstrated the validity of patient satisfaction as an important proxy for health care quality. For example, continuity of care has long been seen as a measure of quality of care. The RAND data demonstrated a clear association between patient satisfaction and continuity of care. For a one-point decrease on a general satisfaction scale, there was a 3.4 percentage increase in the probability of an individual's changing health care providers (Marquis, Davies, and Ware, 1983).

Health status is another well-accepted measure of the quality of care. Hall and others (Cleary, 1988) reviewed articles on the association between health status and satisfaction with care. The majority of the reviewed studies reported positive associations between health status and satisfaction. As health status increased, satisfaction rose as well. Furthermore, other studies have demonstrated that improvement in health is a predictor of improved patient satisfaction. Research is beginning to illuminate the connection between satisfied patients and quality health care (Carmel, 1985; Fleming, 1981).

Commonly Measured Aspects of Satisfaction

Patient satisfaction is commonly measured through surveys that ask patients about their experiences. When patient satisfaction surveys are designed and implemented, both the physical environment and time frame to be addressed must be clearly specified in the questions because both of these components affect how respondents perceive and answer questions. Items addressing the location of care usually fall into one of two categories: outpatient (such as physician offices and clinics) or inpatient (hospitals or other institutions).

Like location of care, the time frame typically falls under one of two headings: global and visit specific. A global time frame refers to a patient's overall experience with a primary care physician (PCP) or specialist, usually limited to the past twelve months. An advantage of using this method is that an understanding of how satisfied patients are with services can be obtained quickly and with limited resources (one or two survey administrations). However, this method also reduces an organization's ability to "drill down" the results to specific encounters and account for seasonal variations in satisfaction. Visit-specific time frames refer to a particular visit, which can be described as the last or most recent date that care was provided. Although this method can be more resource intensive, it does allow for critical examination of results and correlation with services actually received. For example, Pascoe and Attkison (1983) formulated and tested the Evaluation Ranking Scale and found that this measure provided more specific information, was more discriminating, and resulted in significantly lower satisfaction scores overall than did a global measure.

Through thirty years of measuring patient satisfaction, standard items have emerged for the different locations of care and time periods. For outpatient or clinic settings, these include:

- Access to medical care (including specialist and hospitals)
- Technical quality of the doctor
- Communication between the doctor and patient
- Convenience and ease of getting to the physician's office
- Friendliness of the physician and courtesy of the staff
- Overall quality of care

Inpatient satisfaction questionnaires usually focus on the following items (Ross Davies and Ware, 1991):

- Ease of the admission and discharge process
- Skill of doctors
- Information provided by the doctor
- Courtesy of the doctor
- Thoroughness and courtesy of nurses and other hospital staff

Encounter-specific questionnaires measure aspects of care similar to global outpatient or inpatient survey, but use questions tailored to a specific visit rather than the overall experience.

Measurement Issues

How patient satisfaction is measured affects the validity of the data obtained and its acceptability. Measurement issues that are often raised and debated are the choice of response scales, sampling, response bias, convenience of the survey administration to the patient and staff, and reporting of information.

There has long been a debate, which will no doubt continue, concerning which response scale to use when measuring patient satisfaction. Response scales usually contain five or seven categories that the questionnaire respondents can choose from to rate their satisfaction with a certain aspect of care. The more traditional satisfaction rating scales are "very satisfied" to "very dissatisfied" or "strongly agree" to "strongly disagree." For example, a patient is typically asked, "How satisfied are you with . . ." and responds "very satisfied," "somewhat satisfied," "neither satisfied nor dissatisfied," "somewhat dissatisfied," or "very dissatisfied." Although these two scales have been shown to be valid, evidence is growing that a response scale asking patients to rate their experiences from excellent to poor (Excellent, Very Good, Good, Fair, Poor) is a more precise measure of satisfaction and demonstrates superior validity (Ware and Hays, 1988). Regardless of which response scale is used, it is important to use the same scale as much as possible throughout a questionnaire so that comparisons can be made among the different aspects of satisfaction measured by the survey.

Recall bias also affects the validity of satisfaction data. A frequently voiced criticism of data gathered through surveys is how someone can remember what happened three months or a year ago. This is a valid concern that must be considered when collecting satisfaction data. Data gathered through a questionnaire administered immediately after a doctor's visit gives the most precise results because the respondent's memory has not been affected by the passage of time; nevertheless, valid data can be collected retrospectively. Normally this is accomplished by instructing the respondents to answer each question concerning their last visit or about their physician in general. Research has demonstrated that asking individuals to recall information about a visit that occurred two to three months ago does not introduce recall bias (Brown and Adams, 1992).

Response rate is yet another aspect of survey administration that affects the quality and generalizability of satisfaction data. A good response rate (usually over 30 percent of individuals surveyed) ensures a representative cross-section of a physician's or physician group's patient population and minimizes the effect of outliers. The most effective way to guarantee a good response rate is to make the administration of the survey as easy as possible for the patient, physician, and office staff. One way to achieve this is by drawing samples with adequate statistical power to measure significant differences and changes in the population rather than trying to survey an entire population. The appropriate sample size can be determined for a specific population through a power calculation (Zar, 1984), thus reducing the number of surveys needed in order to measure meaningful differences. Surveying the minimum number of patients necessary to obtain meaningful data reduces the amount of intrusion on patients and staff while still obtaining usable results.

Merging demographic and clinical data with satisfaction data can enhance the benefit of the analysis. By adding procedure (CPT–4) and diagnosis (ICD–9 and diagnosis-related groups) data to satisfaction data, differences in satisfaction can be stratified by procedure and diagnosis. Adaptations to medical practice can be made to increase consumer satisfaction with medical procedures and conditions that have historically shown low levels of satisfaction.

Merging clinical data introduces some unique problems that should be clearly thought out before administering the satisfaction questionnaire. Most important, a medical group should address what clinical or demographic data will be useful to merge. By and large, these data will be used to stratify and adjust the satisfaction data, so this goal should drive the decision. Commonly this list includes insurance carrier since the type of insurance and the latitude a patient has in choosing a physician have been shown to influence patient satisfaction (Shmittdiel, Selby, Grumbach, and Quensenberry, 1997); procedure codes because different levels of satisfaction are associated with different procedures; and diagnosis codes because some diagnoses or disorders such as psychiatric disorders generally confer lower levels of satisfaction (Harmon, Ettner, and Dorwart, 1998). The actual merging of data requires that the diagnosis or procedure data be correctly associated with the satisfaction data for a specific encounter. An easy way to achieve this is to use an encounter-specific identification on the patient satisfaction survey and in the clinical or administrative database to guarantee a match between the data sets. If a medical group does not have an electronic database that contains clinical information, the data will have to be abstracted from medical charts. This extra step will make the data matching process immensely more time intensive and expensive.

Using Satisfaction Data to Profile Physicians

John Wennberg and colleagues have demonstrated a significant variation in physician practice patterns (Wennberg, Barnes, and Zubkoff, 1982; Wennberg and Gittelsohn, 1982). This source of variation is the underpinning of physician profiling. By identifying sources of meaningful variation in practice patterns, physicians and physician groups can be profiled to distinguish best practices. Organizations (health plans or group practices) can then provide quality reimbursements to the best practices and implement quality improvement programs targeting the practices that fell short of that mark.

Since its introduction, physician profiling has been largely confined to the examination of economic and clinical efficiency. Economic efficiency refers to a population-based, case-mix-adjusted approach to analyzing the overall financial impact of the manner in which physicians practice medicine. The cost of practice variation is important to both health plans and physicians as they work to define and manage physician reimbursement appropriately and price contracts with each other fairly. Clinical efficiency is usually measured through a disease-specific approach that analyzes the utilization of services for a particular disease, the associated treatment patterns, and outcomes of care across physicians or treatment settings.

Patient satisfaction results increasingly are being used, in addition to utilization and clinical outcome measures, to profile physicians. Health plans and now large group practices are using satisfaction data to supplement existing profiling mechanisms (such as that conducted by Aetna/U.S. Healthcare) or are profiling physicians on the basis of satisfaction results alone (Schlackman, 1989; Hanchak, Schlackman, and Harmon Weiss, 1996).

Following is a description of the steps a group practice must think through to develop a patient satisfaction assessment plan.

A large group practice that has approximately one hundred physicians and ten sites has decided to administer a patient satisfaction survey to determine areas in which improvement is needed to keep patients satisfied. Furthermore, they want to use this information to profile and compare doctors and clinics against their peers so that those whose patients are most satisfied with their services can be acknowledged and those whose patients are least satisfied can improve.

The first decision that the group practice had to make was whether their satisfaction tool should be specific to the last visit or ask globally about the physician an individual sees the most. They chose a questionnaire that asks patients to rate their global experiences with the physician and clinic because they were most concerned with the ongoing relationship of the patient, physician, and clinic. They also decided to mail questionnaires twice a year since this will be less disruptive to the office staff than handing them out in the office and will take into account seasonal variation in responses.

The questionnaire, a variation of the Group Health Association of America's (GHAA) satisfaction questionnaire, can be filled out quickly and has a consistent response scale ("excellent" to "poor"), which facilitates reliable comparisons among different aspects of care. For data entry purposes, they elected to buy a scanning tool, which reduced the administrative resources needed to enter the questionnaires and reduced, if not eliminated, keypunch errors. Finally, they opted to sample a portion of each doctor's patients randomly during each six-month period to reduce the number of patients asked to fill out the questionnaire.

In analyzing the responses, frequencies of all responses for each question were compiled to look for data quality issues. Responses were dichotomized so that "excellent" and "very good" represented satisfaction with that aspect of care and "good," "fair," or "poor" represented dissatisfaction with an aspect of care. The percentage of individuals who were satisfied ("excellent" or "very good") was calculated for each doctor and clinic. Means and standard deviations of these percentages were also calculated for all doctors and clinics. Statistical significance was determined by a chi-square test, and doctors and clinics in the upper and lower quintiles of satisfaction were identified. Results were reported by clinic and physician. Figure 8.1 demonstrates a sample report for the question, "How would you rate the overall quality of care and services you received from your doctor?"

The doctors and the clinic administrators interpreted these reports for quality improvement purposes. The graph in Figure 8.1 plots the percentage of individuals, for each clinic and a specific physician, who rate the overall quality of care and services received from their doctor as being either "excellent" or "very good." Also, the average percentage and the eightieth and twentieth percentiles for the entire group practice were plotted. Each clinic was compared to the mean for the entire group practice. Physicians and clinics that fell above the eightieth percentile were deemed to be "best practices," and those below the twentieth percentile were identified as "worst practices." This type of reporting was done for all aspects of satisfaction measured.

In addition to point estimates, the group practice looked at results over time by using a control chart (see Figure 8.2). Point estimates for each physician or clinic every six months were charted along with the lower (-2 standard deviations) and upper (+2 standard deviations) bounds for the entire survey population. This method allowed the group practice to identify variation in patient satisfaction and see when a clinic or physician was significantly "out of control" for the purpose of quality improvement and process control.

FIGURE 8.1. SAMPLE PATIENT SATISFACTION CHART.

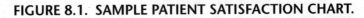

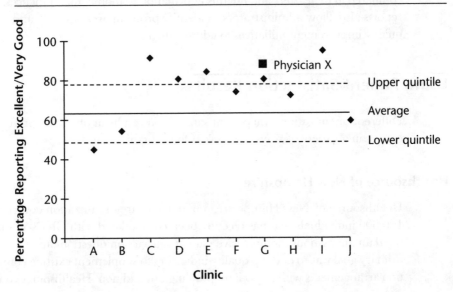

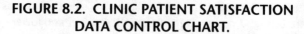

FIGURE 8.2. CLINIC PATIENT SATISFACTION DATA CONTROL CHART.

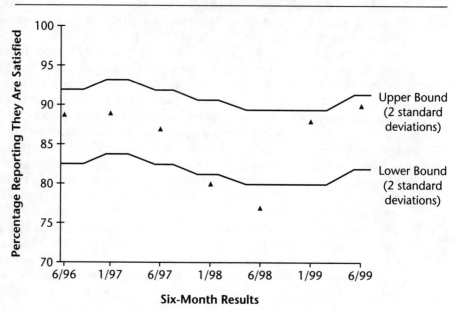

By using these methods of reporting data, physicians can quickly see how they compared to their peers and use this information to modify their practices. These reports also allow administrators to identify problem areas quickly and develop quality improvement initiatives to address them.

Using Patient Satisfaction Results

Different organizations use patient satisfaction results in physician profiling initiatives in a variety of ways. We look at four organizations here.

Healthsource of New Hampshire

Healthsource of New Hampshire, a managed care organization covering over 100,000 individuals that has recently been consolidated with CIGNA, administered an anonymous, nonintrusive patient satisfaction questionnaire by mail. Its primary goal was to develop quality indicators to supplement existing compensation arrangements with physicians (profiling). In addition, Healthsource sought to use satisfaction results to determine whether undercare was an issue in a fiscally conservative environment; support National Committee for Quality Assurance (NCQA) accreditation, Health Plan Employer Data and Information Set (HEDIS) reporting, and other performance measurement initiatives; strengthen network development; and set in place an ongoing quality and statistical process control for quality improvement efforts.

Healthsource's satisfaction questionnaire was short (fewer than twenty-five questions) and easy for patients to complete. It measured the following aspects of satisfaction in respect to the individual's last office visit:

- Length of time to get an appointment
- Amount of time spent waiting in the office
- Length of time spent with the doctor
- Convenience of office hours
- Thoroughness of treatment
- Attention given to what the patient had to say
- Preventive information and advice
- Confidence in the doctor
- Courtesy of doctor and office staff
- Overall satisfaction with the visit

The questionnaires were scannable to minimize keypunch errors and were accompanied by a letter from Healthsource's chief executive officer explaining why the plan was sending this questionnaire, instructions on how to fill it out, and thanking the respondent for choosing to participate. Questionnaires for pediatricians were mailed to the parents or guardians of the child receiving services. Physician identification numbers were preprinted on the questionnaire to reduce errors and administrative hassles.

In order for physicians to be eligible to participate in the patient satisfaction survey, they had to be a primary care physician functioning in a gatekeeper role and serve more than one hundred patients in their panel. Patients of qualifying physicians received questionnaires throughout the year. In order to minimize recall bias, they were surveyed within sixty days of their visit. The objective was to receive at least thirty-five responses per physician per year with a minimum response rate of 30 percent.

An elaborate sampling mechanism was created to gain a representative cross-section of a physician's patients throughout the year and to reduce the number of individuals needed to complete the survey while still being able to make a statistically meaningful comparison among physicians. Twice a month, Healthsource created a data set consisting of new claims for the past two weeks and sent it to the data management center at HCIA. Each physician's claim lag was calculated. The claim lag was predefined to have a minimum value of thirty days and a maximum value of fifty days. This ensured that no individual would receive a questionnaire more than sixty days after the visit. The claim lag procedure ensured that over 90 percent of all encounters for a given physician during each time period were considered in the sampling.

The number of surveys to be sent each administration period for each physician was then calculated. This calculation was based on each physician's historical response rate and the number of administrations left in the current year. The calculation ensured that the distribution of completed questionnaires was evenly distributed throughout the year and that no physician ended the year with too many or too few questionnaires based on the required goal of thirty-five per physician. Members were randomly selected from the available pool of claims for a two-week period to match the number of questionnaires needed for each physician. Patients who had already received a satisfaction questionnaire during the year were excluded from the random sample so no patient was asked to fill out more than one questionnaire per year, even for a different visit.

At the end of the year, multiple analyses were performed. For the specific purpose of physician profiling, frequencies for each physician's and physician group's patients were calculated for each question on the survey and fed back to Healthsource. Beyond frequencies, responses were dichotomized into percentage of individuals reporting "excellent" or "very good." This was done for each physician and compared to the average rate for his or her peer group. Usually physicians in the upper quintile were deemed to have the "best practice" and received a predetermined bonus, which is a percentage of their capitated reimbursement.

The Healthsource example demonstrates a highly evolved data collection methodology that minimizes recall bias, which is common in survey administration. It also illustrates how health plans are using patient satisfaction results to compare physicians, with the ultimate goal being to increase consumer satisfaction with their product (medical care).

Olathe Medical Services

Health plans comprise the largest portion of organizations using patient satisfaction data to profile physicians, but a growing number of multisite group practices are integrating profiling physician and patient satisfaction into their management of medical care. Olathe Medical Services is a group of fifteen outpatient clinics located throughout Kansas that employs approximately four hundred physicians, mostly general practitioners. For a little over a year, the organization has been administering a patient satisfaction questionnaire specifically designed for physician offices. The primary goal for expending the time and effort to administer these questionnaires was to profile physicians and clinics. The profiles generated were used to compare physicians internally to improve quality and grant financial bonuses.

Olathe uses an outpatient satisfaction questionnaire adapted from a consumer satisfaction questionnaire developed by GHAA. It measures the following aspects of satisfaction in respect to an individual's perception of the doctor's office or clinic he or she visited:

- Access to medical care such as specialty and hospital
- The technical quality of the doctor
- Communication between the doctor and patient
- Convenience and ease of getting to the physician's office
- Friendliness of the physician
- Courtesy of the staff
- Overall quality of care received

The outpatient satisfaction questionnaire was originally administered on site to every individual after each visit. This methodology was changed after a few months because it was too cumbersome for the office staff, and many patients were filling out the survey multiple times, which could potentially bias the results. Olathe changed the methodology to a systematic sample, with every third person who walked through the clinic's doors receiving a questionnaire. Although this is not a random sample of patients per doctor, it does not allow much, if any, bias into the sample because of the frequency of administration and the volume of patients.

Pacific Business Group on Health

The most aggressive use of results from satisfaction questionnaires is seen in the application of regional business coalitions—loose alliances of CEOs and upper management from leading industries in a geographic area. Their purpose is to increase contracting power with managed care organizations and in some instances large physician practices. Their goal is to drive down their health care cost while ensuring quality care for their employees and families. The number of these coalitions has steadily risen since the mid-1980s.

The Pacific Business Group on Health (PBGH), one of these groups, encompasses twenty employers providing benefits to over 2.5 million people at a cost of $3 billion annually (Atlantic Information Services, 1996). In 1996 the Pacific Business Group on Health and the Medical Quality Commission conducted a survey to measure patient satisfaction at forty-nine California and nine Pacific Northwest (Oregon and Washington) physician groups. The PBGH's goal was to use this information in contracting and make it available to the public, specifically their employees.

The satisfaction questionnaire was short and easy for patients to complete. It asked individuals to rate the following aspects of care they received from their physician group over the previous year:

- Thoroughness of treatment
- Time with the doctor and staff
- The quality of the specialists
- Whether they waited more than thirty minutes to see a doctor
- Whether they waited more than fifteen days to get an appointment
- Overall satisfaction with the doctor
- Overall quality of care and services

This survey, administered by an independent research firm, was mailed to all employees from the participating companies who went to one of the fifty-eight physician groups. (Not all of the physician groups elected to participate.) Over thirty-one thousand patients responded to the questionnaire.

Although the reporting of satisfaction results was done in a fairly standard way for profiling physicians and physician groups, the scope and means of dissemination were quite radical. The PBGH reported for each physician group the percentage of individuals reporting satisfaction with all areas of the survey by geographic region. Each score was categorized as being significantly above the average or below the average for respondents from that region.

What is unique about PBGH's effort to profile physician groups is how and where this information is dispersed. If the profiling effort is done through a health plan, results are typically distributed internally within the organization and externally to the physicians or administrators of a group practice. PBGH publishes the results on its Web page for public consumption and actively encourages employees to look at the results when they are choosing a doctor or health plan (Pacific Business Group on Health, 1998).

Center for Research in Ambulatory Health Care Administration at the Medical Group Management Association

Group and trade associations have also started to emphasize and promote the use of patient satisfaction results in profiling physicians. As a result of several hundred telephone inquiries of members of the Medical Group Management Association (MGMA) concerning the use of patient satisfaction data in group practices, the Center for Research in Ambulatory Health Care Administration (CRAHCA) and

HCIA have recently entered into a collaboration to facilitate the measurement of patient satisfaction and the compilation of practice profiling or comparisons. As part of this agreement, HCIA provides the Starting Line software package, which optically scans survey cards at a reduced price. CRAHCA provides a standard patient satisfaction survey.

The CRAHCA patient satisfaction tool contains thirty-three questions: questions from the GHAA visit-specific satisfaction questionnaire and the health conditions list from the member satisfaction questionnaire. This survey measures satisfaction with the following items:

- Length of time to get an appointment
- Convenience of office location
- Getting through to the office by telephone
- Time waited at the office
- Time spent with the doctor
- Technical skills and the doctor's personal manner
- The visit overall
- Likelihood of recommending the clinic to family or friends
- A comorbidity checklist

As part of the effort to provide both internal and external profiling capabilities, CRAHCA requested that groups wishing to compare their experiences to external results submit a specific number of survey administrations per physician to HCIA every six months for inclusion into HCIA's National Outcomes Data Warehouse. Groups submitting information to the warehouse will receive regular benchmarking reports comparing their institution to other similar institutions. Since most practice profiling efforts to date have been limited to profiling physicians' satisfaction results within their own organization, the opportunity to create profiles that incorporate practices from different geographic regions, socioeconomic makeup, and patient populations is exciting. From both an operational and research standpoint, the variation in satisfaction should be examined both internal and external to an organization.

Marketing Patient Satisfaction Results

Patient satisfaction data hold value to health care organizations beyond the uses of profiling physicians and assessing health care quality. The growing trend is to use satisfaction results to market a physician's or group of physicians' services to consumers. With the supply of physicians growing, increased patient sophistication, and the entry of for-profit organizations into the marketplace, providers are becoming increasingly interested in marketing patient satisfaction results. They are using their results in capitation negotiation with managed care organizations and to attract new patients.

Patient Satisfaction and the Internet

Health care is about information. The faster that data can be collected, transformed into information, and disseminated, the faster decisions can be made. As a result, we have seen the use of the Internet and World Wide Web by medicine, and health care in general, grow exponentially. Telemedicine and on-line medical charts are becoming common practice in some institutions. For example, clinicians hundreds of miles away from each other are simultaneously viewing the same computed tomography scans for consultation. As the Pacific Business Group on Health has demonstrated, the Web and Internet is an efficient medium for the dissemination of patient satisfaction results to consumers. Beyond basic dissemination of information, the Web is becoming an efficient way to collect patient satisfaction and functional status data. Products already on the market facilitate the automated collection of scanned survey information through Web browsers in a secure environment. The advantages of using the power of the Web are clear: useful information is quickly and easily made available to individuals for incorporation in the decision-making process.

The Future

On a personal level, patient satisfaction has always been important to doctors. The physician-patient relationship is grounded in trust and caring by both parties. The current trends in health care are merely elevating the examination of that relationship to a higher level of scrutiny. Some argue this step should not be taken because it could hurt the personal nature of the physician-patient relationship; others say that it will only strengthen the relationship since physicians and administrators will be able to identify issues with a population approach that they otherwise would have missed on a one-to-one level.

The future holds many advances in the measurement and application of patient satisfaction to physician profiling. The number of health plans, specifically managed care organizations, that are measuring and profiling physicians on the basis of patient satisfaction will increase. The likely driver of their development is attaining and maintaining accreditation with the National Committee for Quality Assurance. Health plans increasingly will apply patient satisfaction results to the profiling of specialists. In the past, patient satisfaction results have been largely confined to profiling of primary care physicians. However, as the health care system grapples with the gatekeeper role, the examination of practice patterns within specialties will increase. Health plans will also expend more resources to develop reimbursement formulas that incorporate satisfaction measurement. The influence that business coalitions have on our health care system will increase and greatly affect the use of satisfaction information. The three most important aspects of health care to industry are whether their employees are able to work or function to their fullest, whether their employees are happy with the medical care they receive, and the cost to employers. Health plans are not going to bite the hand that feeds them; they will increase their responsiveness to industry and consumer groups. Finally, the incidence of physician practices that measure and apply patient satisfaction will increase.

Conclusion

Our health care environment is developing into a population-based and more consumer-driven system, and patient satisfaction has become an important quality-of-care outcome measure. In addition, health plans and group practices commonly use satisfaction data to profile physicians to support the determination of financial incentives. Common aspects of measuring satisfaction include addressing the physical environment and the time frame a patient satisfaction questionnaire refers to. The measurements to consider include a practice's choice of a response scale, recall bias, and the desired response rate. Merging demographic and clinical data with satisfaction data can improve a clinic's satisfaction analysis. This can be achieved by adding insurance carrier, procedure codes, and diagnostic codes to the satisfaction database. In addition to using the satisfaction data in profiling physicians, results increasingly are used to market a physician's or group of physicians' services to consumers and to support contract negotiations with health plans. New Internet-based applications of patient satisfaction tools are available to ease communication, access, and analysis of satisfaction data. In the future, the number of health plans measuring and profiling physicians on the basis of patient satisfaction is going to increase. Many aspects of our health care system will be debated for years to come, but there is one certainty: the consumer will be important.

References

Atlantic Information Services. *A Guide to Patient Satisfaction Survey Instruments: Profile of Patient Satisfaction Measurement Instruments and Their Use by Health Plan, Hospitals, and Insurers.* Washington, D.C.: Atlantic Information Services, 1996.

Brown, J. B., and Adams, M. E. "Patients as Reliable Reporters of Medical Care Process: Recall of Ambulatory Encounter Events." *Medical Care*, 1992, *30*(5), 400–411.

Carmel, S. "Satisfaction with Hospitalization: A Comparative Analysis of Three Types of Services." *Social Science and Medicine*, 1985, *21*, 1243–1249.

Cleary, P. D., and McNeil, B. J. "Patient Satisfaction as an Indicator of Quality Care." *Inquiry*, 1988, *25*, 25–36.

Cronin, C. "Business Coalitions on Health: Their Activities and Impact." *Joint Commissions Journal on Quality Improvement*, 1994, *20*(7), 376–380.

Fleming, G. V. "Hospital Structure and Consumer Satisfaction." *Health Services Research*, 1981, *16*, 43–63.

Hanchak, N. A., Schlackman, N., and Harmon Weiss, S. "U.S. Healthcare's Quality-Based Compensation Model." *Health Care Finance Review*, 1996, *17*(3), 143–159.

Harmon, R. C., Ettner, S. L., and Dorwart, R. A. "The Influence of Psychiatric Disorders on Patients' Ratings of Satisfaction with Health Care." *Medical Care*, 1998, *36*(5) 720–727.

Marquis, M. S., Davies, A. R., and Ware, J. E. "Patient Satisfaction and Change in Medical Care Provider: A Longitudinal Study." *Medical Care*, 1983, *21*(8), 821–829.

Pacific Business Group on Health. [http://www.healthscope.org/pg/pat_sat/prom/p_pat_sat_prom_cc.htm]. 1998.

Pascoe, G. C., and Attkison, C. C. "The Evaluation Ranking Scale: A New Methodology for Assessing Satisfaction." *Evaluation and Program Planning*, 1983, *6*, 335–347.

Ross, C. K., Steward, C. A., and Sinacore, J. M. "A Comparative Study of Seven Measures of Patient Satisfaction." *Medical Care*, 1995, *33*(4), 392–406.

Ross Davies, A., and Ware, J. E. *GHAA Consumer Satisfaction Survey and User's Manual*. Washington, D.C.: Group Health Association of America, 1991.

Schlackman, N. "Integrating Quality Assessment and Physician Incentive Payment." *Joint Commission Journal on Quality Improvement*, 1989, *15*(8), 234–237.

Shmittdiel, J., Selby, J. V., Grumbach, K., and Quensenberry, C. P. "Choice of Personal Physician and Patient Satisfaction in Health Maintenance Organizations." *Journal of the American Medical Association*, 1997, *278*(19), 1596–9.

Ware, J. E., and Hays, R. D. "Methods for Measuring Patient Satisfaction with Specific Medical Encounters." *Medical Care*, 1988, *26*, 393–402.

Wennberg, J. E., Barnes, B. A., and Zubkoff, M. "Professional Uncertainty and the Problem of Supplier-Induced Demand." *Social Science Medicine*, 1982, *16*(7), 811–824.

Wennberg, J. E., and Gittelsohn, A. "Variations in Medical Care Among Small Areas." *Scientific American*, 1982, *246*(4), 120–134.

Williams, S. J., and Torrens, P. R. *Introduction to Health Services*. (4th ed.) Albany, N.Y.: Delmar, 1993.

Zar, J. H. *Biostatistical Analysis*. (2nd ed.) Englewood Cliffs, N.J.: Prentice Hall, 1984.

CHAPTER NINE

TURNING ANALYSIS INTO ACTION

Profiling as a Change Agent

Jay Noren, Robin M. Thibodeau,
Ralph Insinga, Beth Marie Landon

Physician profiling methods are commonly used tools for stimulating physician behavior change toward more effective and efficient care. They are intended to improve physician quality of care and reduce practice variation without compromising patient outcomes.

Physician profiles provide information about actual practice behavior, using epidemiological methods to compare patterns of practice (Shapiro, Lasher, and Bindman, 1993). Rather than using isolated examples to provide peer comparison information to physicians, profiles make direct comparisons of physician performance with that of their colleagues within the practice as well as across practices. This type of feedback is designed to stimulate consensus and enable physicians to make informed decisions on how to treat their patients (Keller, Soule, and Wennberg, 1990). Substantial evidence demonstrates that such feedback produces changes in physicians' practice patterns (Davis, Thomson, and Oxman, 1992; Manus, Werner, and Strub, 1994; Rosenstein, 1996), although conflicting evidence also exists showing no change in physician behavior (Balas and others, 1996). Physician profiling is most effective in influencing physician behavior when combined with other interventions.

Principles of Behavior Change Related to Physician Profiling

A variety of paradigms and corresponding strategies exist that characterize principles of change in physician practice behavior. One often-cited model groups factors influencing clinical practice into predisposing, enabling, and reinforcing factors (Tamblyn and Battista, 1993; Davis, Thomson, and Oxman, 1992). *Predisposing factors* include the practitioner's knowledge and skills, as well as sociodemographic characteristics. *Enabling factors* facilitate the initiation of new behavior. *Reinforcing factors* are those that sustain behavior over time. Design and implementation of successful physician profiling interventions should incorporate all three factors.

Among the several enabling factors most critical to physician behavior change are intensive physician participation in all phases of profiling program development and implementation, timeliness of data, preservation of optimal physician practice autonomy, clear relevance to potential improvement, collegial interaction, and emphasis on positive (incentives) rather than negative (penalties) interventions.

The role of the reinforcer appears to be of particular importance for all paradigms and strategies. Tamblyn and Battista (1993) suggest that reinforcing factors range from remuneration policies to one-on-one feedback with a credible clinical resource or opinion leader. (Chapter Four in this book looked at clinical information sources that can function as reinforcement factors to effective physician profiling systems.) Bandura (1963) proposes that social reinforcers will be effective for most members of a particular group, since group members share many common social experiences. Essentially the physician social system norms serve as incentives or restraints on the individual's decisions and guide or discourage individuals from adopting the behavior (Rogers and Shoemaker, 1971).

This idea is compounded by Rogers and Shoemaker's (1971) proposal in which physicians do not adopt behaviors at the same rate. Change occurs most readily in physicians with the greatest personal and professional ties (Davis and Fox, 1994). A review by Tamblyn and Battista (1993) concluded that physicians in group practice and those with teaching affiliations have better quality-of-care scores than do those in solo practice. These authors also cite a study of drug innovations that found physicians in group practices adopted new drugs more quickly than did those in solo practice.

Several general theories exist on the process of how people change. We modify three such general theories and apply them to physician profiling by creating five stages for tracking the impact of the profiling system on physician behavior change: (1) justification for evaluation of practice, (2) first profiling data review, (3) individual physician reflection on data, (4) physician decision to alter practice, and (5) second profiling data review or confirmation (see Table 9.1). These five stages have counterparts in the general behavior change theories articulated by Geertsma, Parker, and Whitbourne (1982), and Rogers and Shoemaker (1971) and Prochaska and others (1994).

Stage 1: Recognition

The recognition stage must occur in order to convince physicians that collection of profiling data has some value and relevance to their practices. This justification may be stimulated by forces inside the social system in which the physician works or occur out of a perceived need for self-evaluation combined with curiosity. At times motivation may be external to the physicians' social system and occur when outsiders introduce or impose a planned change (Rogers and Shoemaker, 1971). As Table 9.1 shows, the general behavior models of Geertsma, Parker, and Whitbourne (1982) and Prochaska and others (1994) label this stage "priming" and "contemplation," respectively. The Rogers and Shoemaker (1971) model does not have a stage that can be likened to recognition.

Stage 2: First Profile

Once a physician consciously or unconsciously experiences a problem with current practice behavior, the quest to resolve this dilemma commences. In the profiling context this occurs in the first profiling stage, when initial profiling data are collected and analyzed. Rogers and Shoemaker (1971) calls this self-exposure to ideas in accord with one's interests, needs, or existing attitudes "selective exposure." Geertsma, Parker, and Whitbourne (1982) treat this as the second stage in the readiness-to-change continuum, called "focusing," in which participants are seriously thinking about change and are open to information and feedback. Geertsma, Parker, and Whitbourne note that physicians experience "focusing," in which they become aware of an alternative or new practice behavior, in 96 percent of the changes studied. Rogers and Shoemaker (1971) call this stage "knowledge," and Prochaska and others (1994) include it as part of the first stage, "contemplation." For physicians this stage is typically stimulated by informal information such as printed materials, electronic sources (CD-ROM, Internet), or collegial interaction. Alternatively formal continuing medical education (CME) might provide the stimulus.

Stage 3: Reflection

The third profiling stage, *reflection*, labeled "follow-up" in the Geertsma, Parker, and Whitbourne (1982) model, occurred in 68 percent of the physician behavior change studies, leading these authors to describe it as "crucial to the outcome of the change process" (p. 758). They hypothesize that social influences are particularly

TABLE 9.1. THE FIVE STAGES IN GENERAL BEHAVIOR CHANGE

Stages of Behavior Change	Physician Behavior Change		General Behavior Change Theory	
	Physician Profiling Stages: Impact on Behavior Change	Geertsma Theory Stages: Readiness to Change	Rogers and Shoemaker Theory Stages: Innovation-Decision Process	Prochaska and Others' Theory Stages: Readiness to Change
Stage 1	*Recognition:* Physicians realize a significant clinical service delivery problem has emerged in the practice	*Priming:* Feels cognitive dissonance with some aspect of practice behavior		*Precontemplation:* Period when not intending to change
Stage 2	*First Profile:* Individual physician profiles collected and analyzed	*Focusing:* Becomes aware of alternative practice behavior	*Knowledge:* Exposure to the innovation's existence and a basic understanding of its function	*Contemplation:* Intending to change in near future
Stage 3	*Reflection:* Individual physicians review and reflect on data	*Follow-up:* Further thinking about the change occurs, with active efforts to learn more	*Persuasion:* Forms a favorable or unfavorable attitude toward the innovation	*Preparation:* Actively planning change
Stage 4	*Decision:* Individual physicians decide to alter personal practice patterns	*Rationalization:* Solutions are envisioned to practical problems associated with the potential change	*Decision:* Engages in activities that lead to a choice to accept or reject the innovation	*Action:* Overtly making changes
Stage 5	*Confirmation:* Second profiling data review reinforces and confirms the altered physician practice pattern	*Triggering:* Change is implemented after a clear communication regarding its desirability	*Confirmation:* Seeks reinforcement for the innovation decision, but may reverse the decision if exposed to conflicting messages	*Maintenance:* Taking steps to sustain change

important in physician behavior change at this stage, evidenced by data indicating that colleagues comprised 46 percent of the follow-up (or reflection) information stimulus. This conclusion is supported by theories of operant conditioning and imitation, in which the process of acquiring a new behavior can be considerably shortened by the provision of social models (Bandura, 1963). The Rogers and Shoemaker (1971) model coins this stage "persuasion," in which the individual forms a favorable or unfavorable attitude toward the innovation. Prochaska and others (1994) call it "preparation," defined as trying the new behavior once, before adopting the new behavior completely.

Stage 4: Decision

Profiling stage 4, *decision,* defines the transition from researching and evaluating alternative behaviors to actual implementation. Geertsma, Parker, and Whitbourne (1982), Rogers and Shoemaker (1971), and Prochaska and others (1994) call this stage "decision," "rationalization," and "action," respectively, during which the individual engages in activities that lead to a choice to adopt or reject the innovation. Geertsma, Parker, and Whitbourne report "rationalization" in only 21 percent of the physician changes studied.

Stage 5: Confirmation

The final profiling stage, *confirmation,* can be thought of as reinforcement of the behavior change usually based on a second set of profiling data. All three of the theoretical change models include this stage. Our physician profiling model borrows Rogers and Shoemaker's (1971) final stage, confirmation, which they describe as the individual's seeking reinforcement for the innovation decision he or she has made, but which may reverse by exposure to conflicting messages about the innovation. The final stage of Prochaska and others (1994) is "maintenance," the time of continued process use and relapse prevention. Geertsma, Parker, and Whitbourne (1982) call this final stage "triggering," which they characterize as implementing the change after a clear communication regarding its desirability. They note that triggering occurred in 26 percent of the changes studied.

Applications of Profiling in Practice

Physician profiling systems enable health care administrators to gather and analyze a wide variety of information related to their practices. Lomas and Haynes (1988) propose four key strategies to alter clinical practice: patient directed, educational, administrative, and financial. Here we extend the four strategies to five methods for enhancing behavior: feedback to physicians (including patient feedback), physician education, physician participation, administrative policies and procedures, and financial incentives and penalties.

Potential uses of profiling include studies of resource utilization, physician productivity, patient outcomes, and adherence to practice guidelines. The utility of possessing such information, and the profiling system as a whole, is likely to depend on an organization's abilities to channel findings into improved physician and staff performance. These abilities will likely determine the contribution of profiling systems to the twin goals of improving the quality and efficiency of health care (Tompkins, 1996).

Greco and Eisenberg (1993) have identified five methods for influencing physician practice behavior: feedback, education, participation, administrative policies, and financial incentives and penalties. Of these methods, the feedback of profiling results to physicians has been the traditional route for achieving organizational goals in the context of physician profiling. Nevertheless, there is mounting evidence that feedback to physicians may not be sufficient for the full realization of improvements in the health care delivery system (Balas and others, 1996). In fact, recent studies have shown that the use of a combination of these five methods is often preferable to a reliance on any single method for inducing behavioral changes (Greco and Eisenberg, 1993).

Feedback of Profiling Results to Physicians

Efficacy studies of physician profiling feedback have been decidedly mixed, with results ranging from marked improvements in performance to little or no change in behavior. To understand feedback mechanisms better and the determinants of its success as a catalyst for behavioral change, it will be instructive to view several physician profiling case studies.

A study by Evans, Hwang, and Nagarajan (1995) examined the use of physician profiling in reducing the length of stay (LOS) of patients in a major hospital. Their study focused on a comparison of hospital medical records over a three-year period subdivided into pre- and postprofiling periods. Results were compared within diagnosis-related groups (DRGs), corresponding to similar instances of patient care, while controlling for the severity level of individual cases based on the five-point scale of the Medical Illness Severity Grouping System (MedisGroups). MedisGroups admission severity scores were based on detailed clinical data from patient medical records and ranged from 0, indicating no abnormal findings, to 4, in cases where organ failure occurred. A separate morbidity indicator, ranging from 1 (high) to 3 (low), was also used for patients who remained in the hospital beyond a specified number of days. The specific time chosen for morbidity evaluation is influenced by the incidence of surgery (Thomas and Ashcraft, 1991). Severity and morbidity scores were intended to reduce randomness effects and provide additional insight into cost variation based on LOS. The data analyzed consisted of 24,396 patients, 379 physicians, and 456 DRGs. Following the initial profiling period, department heads met quarterly with individual physicians to review statistics such as the average patient LOS and average hospital charges, as well as alternative patient treatment policies. The data compared each physician's care, within those DRGs comprising at least 15 patients, to that of all other hospital physicians in the same DRG. In this way, a benchmark was established relating each physician's pattern of care to the average cost and LOS of other physicians within the same DRG. In addition, physicians received reports by DRG for each group in which at least one patient was treated.

Following the initial profiling period, the percentage of physicians who achieved the initial LOS benchmark increased from 61.8 percent to 66.4 percent. The benchmark was then adjusted to reflect the new LOS average for each DRG. In the next profiling period, the number of physicians achieving the adjusted LOS benchmark rose from 60.4 percent to 64.8 percent. Results in both periods were highly significant and support the conclusion that direct feedback of profiling data to physicians can significantly reduce the average length of stay of hospital patients and thereby achieve a reduction in the cost of patient care. The study also revealed that profiling had the greatest impact on physicians who initially did not achieve the benchmark and treated patients classified at a level of medium severity.

In the first case, researchers found little or no impact on the behavior of physicians who initially achieved the LOS benchmark, while significant improvement was made among those who initially failed to achieve the standard. This result may be interpreted to mean that physicians above the benchmark felt satisfied with their performance and faced no stimulus to make further improvements, while those below the benchmark responded to pressures to improve performance. An instrument for achieving total quality improvement across all physicians may therefore require the use of different presentation methods to different physicians based on individual performance. For instance, data for physicians who achieved the benchmark might be compared to those of the top 10 percent or 25 percent of physicians or a target reduction of LOS based on a physician's prior performance. Thus, practices may wish to experiment with different types of feedback to optimize results.

In the second case, the greatest reductions in LOS occurred in cases where patients' diagnoses were of medium severity. This result reflects the fact that as case severity increases, the physician's ability to influence the outcomes of patient treatment generally decreases. This is a relevant factor when deciding the types of cases to profile and appropriate expectations for physician behavior change. For instance, even if profiling will not improve patient care in the area of LOS for severe cases, it might still be of value in allowing physicians to compare the outcomes of different treatments or be used to influence other variables such as the number of procedures ordered. As a final result, it is likely that the comparison of actual dollar cost data for hospital charges, in addition to LOS data, strengthened the effectiveness of profiling efforts. Given the rapid change in medical costs and the complexity of such calculations at the individual physician level, information on the actual dollar cost of services performed may highlight the importance of cost containment to physicians unaware of their actual impact on health care costs (Ramoska, 1998).

Numerous other case studies show a positive impact of feedback to physicians in attaining organizational goals. For instance, recent studies have shown that feedback is successful in the reduction of laboratory use by emergency physicians, the number of medications prescribed to outpatients, hospital charges for hip replacement surgery, and increased compliance with cancer screening guidelines (Evans, Hwang, and Nagarajan, 1995; Ramoska, 1998; Johnson and Martin, 1996; McPhee, Bird, Jenkins, and Fordham, 1989). It is notable that in several cases, physician feedback has succeeded in attaining results without the need for developing new procedures or educating physicians regarding specific practice behavior. In its purest form, feedback seems to gain its effectiveness by drawing on the innate competitive nature of physicians and a desire to maintain a high standard of care through continuous cost and quality improvements. Also, even without an explicit link to compensation, physicians realize that their reputation may be influenced by physician profiling results, providing an additional stimulus for behavioral change (Evans, Hwang, and Nagarajan, 1995).

Among the less favorable evaluations of profiling feedback is a meta-analysis by Balas and others (1996) that assessed twelve prior studies of feedback impact on physicians' practice behavior. The results showed that ten of the twelve studies analyzed ascribed a positive direction to the impact of feedback based on physician profiling. However, the overall magnitude of the feedback effect was quite modest. Balas and others concluded that peer comparison feedback is influential in only a small portion of overall physician cases and that the potential cost savings are unlikely to exceed the costs of profiling for most clinical procedures. These findings are not inherently inconsistent with the successful application of physician profiling. For instance, we note that the positive influence of profiling feedback could be enhanced by combining other types of quality improvement interventions as well as further research into care processes. Before examining the other options for complementing feedback, it will be useful to review several factors that might boost the success of profiling feedback in achieving organizational goals.

First, it is important to consider the timeliness of feedback. Physicians naturally have greater difficulty in applying feedback results if there is a considerable time lapse between its occurrence and the opportunity for implementation. Improved feedback effectiveness might result from providing information or recommending specific clinical actions at the actual time of decision making through a set of reminders (such as a printed note on the patient's encounter form) (Balas and others, 1996). Shapiro, Lasher, and Bindman (1993) found reminders to be extremely effective in influencing clinical decision making.

Second, the ability of the physician to control the variable being measured should be an important criterion for analysis. For instance, when the physician relies heavily on other support staff or specialists, the total number of procedures ordered may be of greater relevance to the physician than the total charges incurred. In some cases the results of physician profiling data may indicate inefficiencies related to the performance of support staff or administration, and careful distinctions must therefore be made in interpreting results.

Third, physicians must be convinced of the need for improvement within their practice (Greco and Eisenberg, 1993). In one program in which feedback was provided, physicians failed to change their patterns for drug prescriptions to outpatients because they were not convinced that less costly medications were effective (Hershey, Goldberg, and Cohen, 1988).

Fourth, financial incentives should be consistent with the goals of profiling feedback. For example, based on profiling results, a physician might be advised to reduce the number of procedures performed while at the same time being compensated on a fee-for-service basis, which would be inconsistent with the profiling goals and thus discourage the desired behavior.

Fifth, profiling should not place physicians at risk for malpractice claims from practice changes. If profiling results lead to restrictions on access to patient services, those changes must clearly coincide with quality improvement rather than just cost controls. Otherwise physician malpractice concerns will become major barriers to effectiveness.

Sixth, profiling feedback should remain sensitive to patient preferences and underlying personality traits of physicians in order to achieve optimal positive impact in response to feedback (Epstien, 1991). Careful consideration of patient satisfaction and physician culture will pay large dividends in feedback impact.

All of these factors add considerable complexity to the task of motivating changes in physician behavior. To improve medical care through profiling, it may be necessary to supplement direct feedback with other forms of intervention. The remainder of this section examines the applicability of four other tools for influencing physician behavior.

Physician Education Programs

Targeted educational materials can effectively complement the feedback of profiling results. These materials will help physicians to take advantage of profiling data through specific improvements in the quality and efficiency of their practice. Although education programs can be applied to a wide variety of situations, they are particularly warranted in supplementing profiling feedback in several specific cases.

First, physicians may not fully trust recommendations provided by others (such as health care administrators) that advocate change in specific clinical behaviors—for example, the prescription of less costly drugs, adoption of a new surgical procedure, or introduction of a new examination technique. Many physicians rely primarily on their own experience or colleagues' recommendations in deciding whether to adopt new techniques or interventions (Greer, 1988). They may therefore be more favorably influenced by the presentation of scientific data from a trusted source regarding the impact of practice changes on the quality and efficiency of medical care. (Specific information on appropriate mechanisms can found in Chapter Four.) The process of formal CME, in response to profiling data, has been successfully provided in a number of settings. One approach to CME involves the selection of trusted opinion leaders from within the medical group practice who are then trained externally and return to practices to educate their colleagues. This formula has been used successfully in reducing the rate of cesarean section births (Soumerai and Avorn, 1990). A similar approach may also be taken in which medical leaders receive practice guidelines, which they then distribute to their colleagues. The fact that these guidelines are received from and endorsed by respected members of the medical group yielded dramatic changes in a study of the perioperative use of antibiotics (Everitt and others, 1990).

Second, physician profiling may uncover variations in practice performance that indicate the need for remedial medical education. For example, based on patient outcome data from profiling, it may be decided that certain data aspects of physician X's performance of hip replacement surgery deviate significantly from that of his or her peers. It may then be decided to offer remedial education to assist this physician in achieving a given benchmark level of performance. Rather than sanctioning the physician, the opportunity to receive this education can be viewed as a value-added alternative for both the physician and the organization. This type of education, sometimes referred to as academic detailing, has been effective in influencing physician behavior in virtually every study in which it has been used (Greco and Eisenberg, 1993). Using profiling data analyses, U.S.

Healthcare, a health care organization, provided a refresher course to physicians covering breast exam techniques. Tests given before and after the course revealed a fourfold increase in average ability to detect breast masses. An additional test six months later found that physicians had retained that ability (Schlackman, 1996). A key disadvantage to remedial education is that it is a relatively costly and labor-intensive intervention.

A third educational complement to profiling occurs when neither administrators nor physicians can identify a suitable plan of attack for controlling costs without compromising quality. This is more likely a factor when profiling data make comparisons across rather than within medical groups. Education programs and materials may help to identify and eliminate unnecessary services, choose the less costly of equally effective alternative forms of care, and select preventive services that will act as cost-saving devices over the long run (Shapiro, Lasher, and Bindman, 1993).

In general, educational interventions have been most effective when the curriculum targets specific aspects of behavior rather than merely presenting the current state of scientific knowledge in a particular area (White, Albenese, Brown, and Caplan, 1985). For instance, one study found that the provision of educational memoranda advocating the use of a specific diagnostic test for thyroid treatment resulted in widespread adoption of the technique and a 7 percent reduction in laboratory charges for thyroid testing (Schectman, 1991). Even so, education has not always been effective. Physicians may choose to ignore educational guidelines due to contradicting financial incentives, fears of malpractice litigation, patient preferences, or lack of necessary equipment (Greco and Eisenberg, 1993). Furthermore, some physicians, accustomed to a high degree of autonomy, may resent the interference of both education and feedback. These interventions can seem threatening if they are seen as purely external forces, over which the physician lacks input and control, that mandate significant practice changes. Increasing physician participation in decision making can reduce these concerns.

Physician Participation in Decision Making

Increasing physician participation in the application of profiling results can serve a number of useful purposes, from raising physician support for the profiling system to assisting in the development of strategic goals. For a profiling system to function properly, physicians must regard the results as both credible and useful to their practice. Also, physicians will generally oppose reforms they perceive as threatening to their livelihood, self-esteem, sense of competence, or autonomy (Greco and Eisenberg, 1993). Increasing the level of physician participation in the discussion of results and development of guidelines and policies for change can therefore increase both the initial acceptance of the profiling system and the implementation of practice changes. This is particularly important when profiling results suggest the need for a significant change in practice behavior across a large segment of the physician population. Improvements in the design of the profiling system itself, such as data-gathering techniques, can also be developed through physician participation (Shapiro, Lasher, and Bindman, 1993).

Analogous to the case for education, there may be some instances in which the proper interpretation of profiling results is of considerable debate, particularly when there is controversy over the balance between the cost and quality of care. Physician input, aided by clinical experience, is essential to resolving serious issues and designing tailor-made solutions to the unique needs and goals of each organization. This participation in decision making may occur at the diagnostic group, medical group, or regional level. The Maine Medical Assessment Foundation represents an example of success within the last approach. Groups of physicians were organized to study practice variations that focused on utilization patterns that substantially exceeded target levels. The physicians were able to respond to profiling data by identifying reasonable target rates that did not compromise the quality of patient care. When they reported back to their individual medical groups, these rates of usage fell significantly and with substantial cost savings (Keller, Chapin, and Soule, 1990).

Appropriateness studies represent a suitable complement to physician profiling that allows for greater physician participation in decision making. These studies define clinical indications for which a service is appropriate, inappropriate, or equivocal. These classifications are determined by a group of physician experts using literature reviews and group discussions. Appropriateness studies have concluded that a third of carotid endarterectomies and 17 percent of coronary angiograms and endoscopies were performed under inappropriate circumstances (Chassin, 1989).

Ideally, profiling systems should involve physicians at all stages of development: initial design, data review and interpretation, system quality improvement, dissemination of results to practicing physicians, and design of appropriate intervention measures. Unfortunately the added costs in terms of time and expense of increasing physician involvement in these processes have often limited the realization of the full benefits of physician participation.

Administrative Policies and Their Impact on Physician Behavior

Despite the value of feedback, education, and participation in motivating positive behavioral change among physicians, conflicting factors may inhibit the effectiveness of these forms of intervention. As a concrete example, consider a medical group in which physicians are compensated on a purely fee-for-service basis. Suppose after controlling for factors such as diagnostic group, severity, and patient age that there remains wide variation among physicians in the number of procedures performed. Physicians urged to reduce the number of procedures performed will face a conflict of interest given the financial disincentives. In these cases, the use of administrative policies such as preauthorization for specialty referrals, laboratory tests, and procedures may be an appropriate mechanism for accomplishing organizational goals. The evaluation of procedure or resource utilization is thus transferred from the practicing physician to a medical director, administrative review, or other review committee process (Kerr and others, 1995). In more serious deviations from the norm, profiling results may indicate risky patterns of behavior, highlighting the need for more serious administrative procedures such as the application of legal, regulatory, or institutional policy interventions.

There are several reasons for limiting the scope of administrative policies resulting from profiling results to special cases. First, organizations should avoid unnecessarily creating bureaucratic red tape that will ultimately impede efficiency. The addition of new personnel or delegation of greater responsibilities to existing personnel may also defeat the purpose of cost containment. Second, mechanisms such as preauthorization or other stringent rules represent a limiting factor on physician autonomy. If these policy prescriptions dominate the response from profiling efforts, physicians may quickly lose their enthusiasm and support for the profiling process. Thus, physician participation in the decision to develop administrative rules and guidelines can be crucial to their successful implementation. Administrative approaches succeed most often when physician groups themselves decide on the types of services that require preauthorization or other methods, based on profiling results of utilization patterns. For instance, the physician group might decide that a physician gatekeeper referral to a cardiothoracic surgeon requires preauthorization but that obstetrician referrals do not (Kerr and others, 1995). Third, the direct effect on patient outcomes of administrative interventions must be well understood by the physicians affected in order to achieve positive practice changes.

The literature on the effectiveness of administrative policies in achieving results is mixed. Simple changes, such as simplifying order forms to reflect suggested dosing intervals for antibiotics and eliminating certain diagnostic tests from order forms, have been successful (Avorn and Soumerai, 1983). More complex measures have been less effective or of unknown benefit (Greco and Eisenberg, 1993).

Financial Incentives and Penalties

Creating financial incentives and penalties to support physician profiling results is perhaps the most controversial and least researched complement to providing feedback. Although there is strong evidence that physicians respond to financial measures, their application is substantially complicated by issues involving the perceived impact on quality of care provided and by the degree of physician input and support of such changes. For these reasons, organizations may wish to pursue other methods for influencing physician behavior before experimenting with complex financial interventions. Financial incentives and penalties can be applied at the medical group, diagnostic group, or individual physician level, depending on the specific results of the profiling data.

At the medical group level, profiling results compared between similar organizations might reveal significant differences in physician productivity. Studies have documented the positive effects of financial incentives (such as fee-for-service compared to other compensation methods) on physician production levels using measures like patient volume and procedures performed (Conrad and others, 1996). However, an organization contemplating changing physician compensation methods in response to profiling data should proceed with much caution. These decisions must confront the complex trade-offs between physician productivity, efficiency, quality of care, patient satisfaction, and other important factors before implementing change. Any changes among alternative financial incentives must be accompanied by vigilant monitoring to prevent undesirable outcomes in patient care. The same vigilance applies to economic incentive for patients. In some cases, the pattern of physician practice may reflect patient preferences rather than physician behavior. The RAND Health Insurance Experiment demonstrated such effects by revealing that providing economic incentives to patients, such as copayments and deductibles, can substantially reduce utilization in these instances. However, patients are often unable to discriminate between appropriate and inappropriate care, and such economic incentive for patients might negatively affect quality (Sui and others, 1986).

At the diagnostic group level, financial bonuses may be awarded based on physicians' achieving or exceeding a given benchmark target. These benchmarks may reflect an external standard, some average for the diagnostic group, or some fixed level of improvement based on each physician's prior level of performance. Again, continuous quality improvement must reflect both physician practice patterns and patient outcomes. Although information exists on the use of these types of bonuses by HMOs, there is a dearth of information pertaining to initiatives by medical groups. Nevertheless, the results may be transferable.

U.S. Healthcare represents a prime example of the active use of financial incentives. Its physicians receive capitated payments, based on patient age, sex, and a burden-of-illness factor that acts as a risk adjustment mechanism. Beyond the base salary, the HMO gathers profiling data on a variety of measures to make peer comparisons for determining performance bonuses. These bonuses offer up to a 3 percent increase above basic capitated rates for superior performance on each relevant performance measure. This system of incentives has been credited with improvements in the areas of mammography screening, colorectal cancer screening, pneumococcal and influenza immunization, and patient satisfaction. Financial incentives may also be supplemented with education, to assist physicians in achieving targets (Schlackman, 1996).

At the individual physician level, practitioners may be singled out for improvement in a specific area of their practice, based on profiling data, and be assigned a unique bonus or penalty formula to prompt improvement in that particular aspect of patient care. A serious problem with honing in financial incentives at this microlevel may be the perceived arbitrariness of its application to individual members of the medical group. Thus, for reasons of avoiding internal friction alone, this option is unlikely to be viable for most practices.

The current climate favors the choice of financial incentives over penalties. The highly negative connotation of penalties is likely to sour physician support for such initiatives at changing care practices. Also, even though penalties and incentives can be designed to be economically equivalent, the perceived loss of revenue arising from financial penalties has the potential for reducing physician satisfaction and negatively affecting patient care. Financial incentives resulting from profiling efforts can lead to greater support for the profiling system itself, as well as providing the impetus for practice change.

The overall use of financial incentives as instruments for influencing physician behavior remains a topic of considerable debate. Even if all other options for motivating practice change were exhausted, conflicts of interest relating to the quality of patient care call into question the use of financial incentives. Profiling data that focus on patient outcomes, patient satisfaction, and other measures of the quality of health care may provide a suitable means for calibrating the proper degree to which financial incentives should be implemented.

Although providing physician feedback is still the dominant method in use, research has shown that a combination of methods is often necessary to harness the full benefits of physician profiling. Specific case studies and examples illustrate practical applications as well as interactions between methods. The ultimate rewards of profiling systems, in terms of cost savings and improvements in the quality of physician care, are likely to depend on health care administrators' abilities to select and implement the appropriate blend of these techniques.

Conclusion

Several classical theories of learning give insight into changing physician behavior with physician profiling systems (Geertsma, Parker, and Whitbourne, 1982; Rogers and Shoemaker, 1971; Prochaska and others, 1994). However, a new paradigm has been developed specific to physician profiling, identifying the key position that physician profiling occupies in the longer, multistage process of achieving improvements in physician practice. This model shows physicians progressing along a pathway toward behavior change starting with problem recognition and proceeding through distinct phases of profiling analysis, reflection on results, resolution to alter practice patterns, and confirmation and reinforcement of behavior change through subsequent profiling.

Although providing feedback of results to physicians can provide a strong stimulus for achieving desired results, it alone may not be sufficient for organizations to realize fully the potential of physician profiling. Other interventions such as education, participation, administrative rules, and financial incentives may be necessary to ensure that physicians advance successfully through the stages of behavior change. Regardless of the methods ultimately chosen, physician profiling should be approached from the perspective that it is a means to improving patient care and not an end in itself. Physicians and administrators who maintain a strong vision of and dedication to efficient and quality health care will reap the rewards of physician profiling systems.

References

Austin, S. M., Balas, E. A., Mitchell, J. A., and Eigman, B. G. "Effect of Physician Reminders on Preventive Care: Meta-analysis of Randomized Clinical Trials." *Journal of American Medical Association*, Symposium supplement, 1994, 121–124.

Avorn, J., and Soumerai, B. "A New Approach to Reducing Sub-Optimal Drug Use." *Journal of the American Medical Association*, 1983, *250*, 1752–1753.

Balas, E. A., and others. "Effect of Physician Profiling on Utilization: A Meta-Analysis of Randomized Clinical Trials." *Journal of General Internal Medicine*, 1996, *11*, 584–590.

Bandura, A. *Social Learning and Personality Development. The Socio-Behavioristic Approach: Principles of Learning.* Austin, Tex.: Holt, Rinehart and Winston, 1963.

Chassin, M. R. *The Appropriateness of Selected Medical and Surgical Procedures: Relationships to Geographic Variations.* Ann Arbor, Mich.: Health Administration Press, 1989.

Conrad, D. A., and others. "Physician Compensation Models in Medical Group Practice." *Journal of Ambulatory Care Management*, 1996, *19*(4), 18–27.

Davis, D. A., and Fox, R. D. *The Physician as Learner.* Chicago: American Medical Association, 1994.

Davis, D. A., Thomson, M. A., and Oxman, A. D. "Evidence for the Effectiveness of CME." *Journal of American Medical Association*, 1992, *268*(9), 1111–1117.

Epstien, A. "Changing Physician Behavior." *Archives of Internal Medicine*, 1991, *151*, 2147–2149.

Evans, J. H., Hwang, Y., and Nagarajan, N. "Physicians' Response to Length of Stay Profiling." *Medical Care*, 1995, *33*(11), 1106–1119.

Everitt, D. E., and others. "Changing Surgical Antimicrobial Prophylaxis Practices Through Education Targeted at Senior Department Leaders." *Infection Control Hospital Epidemiology*, 1990, *11*, 578–583.

Geertsma, R. H., Parker, R. C., and Whitbourne, S. K. "How Physicians View the Process of Change in Their Practice Behavior." *Journal of Medical Education*, 1982, *57*, 752–761.

Greco, P., and Eisenberg, J. "Changing Physicians' Practices." *New England Journal of Medicine*, 1993, *329*(17), 1271–1274.

Greer, A. L. "The State of the Art Versus the State of Science: The Diffusion of New Medical Technologies into Practice." *International Journal of Technology Assessment Health Care*, 1988, *4*, 5–26.

Hershey, C. O., Goldberg, H. I., and Cohen, D. I. "The Effect of Computerized Feedback Coupled with a Newsletter upon Outpatient Prescribing Charges: A Randomized Controlled Trial." *Medical Care*, 1988, *26*, 88–93.

Johnson, C. C., and Martin, M. "Effectiveness of a Physician Education Program in Reducing Consumption of Hospital Resources in Elective Total Hip Replacement." *Southern Medical Journal*, 1996, *89*(3), 282–289.

Keller, R. B., Chapin, A. M., and Soule, D. N. "Informed Inquiry into Practice Variations: The Maine Medical Assessment Foundation." *Quality Assurance Health Care*, 1990, *2*(1), 69–75.

Keller, R. B., Soule, D. N., and Wennberg, J. E. "Dealing with Geographic Variations in the Use of Hospitals: The Experience of the Maine Medical Assessment Foundation Orthopaedic Study Group." *Journal of Bone and Joint Surgery*, 1990, *72A*(9), 1286–1293.

Kerr, E. A., and others. "Managed Care and Capitation in California: How Do Physicians at Financial Risk Control Their Own Utilization?" *Annals of Internal Medicine*, 1995, *123*(7), 500–504.

Lomas, J., and Haynes, R. B. (1988). "A Taxonomy and Critical Review of Tested Strategies for the Application of Clinical Practice Recommendations: From 'Official' to 'Individual' Clinical Policy." *Implementing Preventative Services*, 1988, *4*, 77–94.

Manus, D. A., Werner, T. R., and Strub, R. J. "Using Measurement and Feedback to Reduce Health Care Costs and Modify Physician Practice Patterns." *Top Health Care Financing*, 1994, *21*(1), 73–89.

McPhee, S. J., Bird, J. A., Jenkins, C. N., and Fordham, D. "Promoting Cancer Screening: A Randomized Controlled Trial of Three Interventions." *Archives of Internal Medicine*, 1989, *149*, 1866–1872.

Prochaska, J. O., and others. "Stages of Change and Decisional Balance for 12 Problem Behaviors." *Health Psychology*, 1994, *13*(1), 39–46.

Ramoska, E. A. "Information Sharing Reduces Laboratory Use by Emergency Physicians." *American Journal of Emergency Medicine*, 1998, *16*(1), 34–36.

Rogers, E. M., and Shoemaker, F. F. *Communication of Innovations: A Cross Cultural Approach.* New York: Free Press, 1971.

Rosenstein, A. H. "Provider Profiling: Improving Outcomes of Care." *Journal of Outcomes Management*, 1996, *3*(2), 10–17.

Schectman, J. M. "Effect of Education and Feedback on Thyroid Function Testing Strategies of Primary Care Clinicians." *Archives of Internal Medicine*, 1991, *151*, 2163–2166.

Schlackman, N. "How One Health Plan Gets Doctors to Improve." *Medical Economics*, 1996, *2*(12), 237–239.

Shapiro, D. W., Lasher, R. D., and Bindman, A. B. "Containing Costs While Improving Quality of Care: The Role of Profiling and Practice Guidelines." *Annual Review Public Health*, 1993, *14*, 219–241.

Soumerai, S. B., and Avorn, J. "Principles of Education Outreach to Improve Clinical Decision Making." *Journal of the American Medical Association*, 1990, *263*, 549–556.

Sui, A. L., and others. "Inappropriate Use of Hospitals in a Randomized Trial of Health Insurance Plans." *New England Journal of Medicine*, 1986, *315*(20), 1259–1266.

Tamblyn, R., and Battista, R. "Changing Clinical Practice: Which Interventions Work?" *Journal of Continuing Education in the Health Professions*, 1993, *12*, 273–288.

Thomas, J. W., and Ashcraft, M. L. "Measuring Severity of Illness: Six Severity Systems and Their Ability to Explain Cost Variations." *Inquiry*, 1991, *28*, 39.

Tompkins, C. P. "Physician Profiling in Group Practices." *Journal of Ambulatory Care Management*, 1996, *19*(4), 28–39.

White, C. W., Albenese, M. A., Brown, D. D., and Caplan, R. M. "The Effectiveness of Continuing Medical Education in Changing the Behavior of Physicians Caring for Patients with Acute Myocardial Infarction: A Controlled Randomized Trial." *Annals of Internal Medicine*, 1985, *102*, 686–692.

INDEX

A

Academic detailing, 147

Access: case example study of, 91–96; cost and utilization data for determining, 113–114

Accountability: demands for, *xix, xxxiii;* levels of physician, 24

Accreditation: data required for, 18; patient satisfaction data for, 129, 134

Action stage, 140, 141

Acuity Index Method (AIM), 67

Acuity levels: establishing, in case-mix adjustment, 26, 72; establishing, with ICD-9 codes, 21, 29–30

Ad hoc reference systems, 18

Adams, M. E., 124, 136

Adjusted Clinical Groups (ACGs), 68–69, 73–77, 83; background and development of, 30*n*.2, 83*n*.2; bias susceptibility in, 74–75; classification of Medicaid well and ill with, 75, 76; classification of PPO and HMO groups with, 75, 77;

data sources for, 74; distributor of, 30*n*.2, 83*n*.2; illness burden values for, 77; morbidity level aggregation of, 76–77; reliance of, on diagnosis codes, 26; sample size for, 75, 76–77; studies on, 75–77; version 3.0, 74; version 4.03, 74

Adjusted Diagnostic Groups (ADGs), 74

Adjusting for severity of illness, 37–38, 40, 115–116. *See also* Case mix adjustment

Administrative data: advantages of, 38–39; case mix adjustment based on, 72, 74, 77; limitations of, for specialist profiling, 26; use of, studies on, *xxiii–xxiv;* variations in, 97–98. *See also* Claims data; Enrollment and eligibility data

Administrative policies, 148–149

Aetna/U.S. Healthcare, 126

Agency for Health Care Policy and Research (AHCPR), 48

Aggregate Condition Categories (ACCs), 78

Alabama, diabetes care study in, *xxiii*

Albenese, M. A., 147, 154

All patient refined diagnosis-related groups (APR-DRGs), 39, 66–67

Ambulatory Care Groups (ACGs), 68, 115, *xxiii. See also* Adjusted Clinical Groups

Ambulatory case mix adjusters, 67

American College of Surgeons, 44

American Medical Association (AMA), 47

Analysis, data. *See* Data analysis

Angina, 37

Appleby, C., 119, 120

Appropriateness studies, 148

Art aspect of medicine, 33–34

Arthritis treatment, 58–60

Ashcraft, M. L., 143, 154

Assumptions about physician behavior: in example of length of stay by admitting physicians in group practice for pneumonia patients, 89–91; in example of patient access report for family practice physicians, 91–96; incorrect, 89–96